AN INTRODUCTION TO APPLIANCE MAKING IN CHIROPODY

An Introduction to
APPLIANCE MAKING
IN CHIROPODY

by

T. THEODORE COATES, M.Ch.S., S.R.Ch.

LECTURER IN APPLIANCES, CHELSEA SCHOOL OF CHIROPODY,
PADDINGTON TECHNICAL COLLEGE

Foreword by Lord Amulree, M.D., F.R.C.P.
President, The Society of Chiropodists

LONDON
THE ACTINIC PRESS LIMITED
13, Tottenham Street, W.1

FIRST PUBLISHED BY
THE ACTINIC PRESS LIMITED
13 TOTTENHAM STREET, LONDON, W.1
IN 1965

MADE AND PRINTED IN GREAT BRITAIN BY
THE GARDEN CITY PRESS LIMITED
LETCHWORTH, HERTFORDSHIRE

CONTENTS

CONTENTS

LIST OF ILLUSTRATIONS

7

FOREWORD

THE successful prevention of painful deformities of the feet is one of the most important aims of all who practise chiropody. Mr. Coates has prepared a book which is full of valuable information of how, by means of simple and ingenious appliances which can be prepared by any practising chiropodist, these disabilities can be prevented or, if this is no longer possible, can be successfully treated. Such a book is bound to be of value to all who are engaged in the profession of chiropody and should find an honoured place wherever disease and disability of the feet is cared for.

August 1964   AMULREE
                         President, Society of Chiropodists

AUTHOR'S NOTE

THE purpose of this book is to outline some of the basic techniques used in making appliances. To this end, pads with differing functions—protection, correction and cushioning—are discussed with a view to amplifying the alternative approaches, and no attempt is made to claim that either the pads themselves or the techniques employed are the only answers to the problems posed. Where a technique is first introduced in the text, it is discussed in considerable detail in relation to one appliance, so that where the same basic method is applied as part of a process of producing a different appliance later on the detail is omitted. Time being a valuable commodity to the practitioner, sound planning of the various stages of appliance-making is essential; as adhesives at one stage are drying so there occurs the opportunity to proceed with another stage. There is no doubt that the intelligent application of appliances in management of cases enhances the value of the work of the chiropodist in his community and to his patient almost immeasurably, and if this book contributes to the advance of the profession in its role of giving a sound foundation on which to build, it will have achieved its object.

I am indebted to Mr. P. J. Read, F.Ch.S., Head of the Chelsea School of Chiropody, for his counsel, advice and encouragement; to Mr. D. Ames, M.Ch.S., Head of the Cardiff School of Chiropody, and to my colleague Mr. J. W. J. Turvey, M.Ch.S., for reading the manuscript and for their helpful comments and suggestions. My grateful thanks also to the many others who in various ways have made this work possible.

London, 1964   T. THEODORE COATES

CHAPTER I

INTRODUCTION TO APPLIANCE MAKING

In the sense in which the subject is to be dealt with here, an appliance is a semi-permanent pad or stiffener which is either removable and placed on the foot, removable and placed in the shoe, or incorporated permanently in the shoe as a modification. Made of more durable materials than felt, Z.O. strapping, tubular bandage and so on, it may be designed to redistribute pressure over an area, to cushion a specific zone, or to re-align the foot to its proper functional position; in short, it can perform most of (and occasionally more than) the functions of adhesive padding whilst at the same time obviating any necessity for an adhesive mass to be in contact with the skin for lengthy periods with resultant possible maceration. At the same time, it does not usually replace the use of conventional padding entirely, as it cannot give the skin traction achieved by strapping, thus it follows that it is necessary to bring the condition under control first with conventional adhesive materials until such time as as much improvement as possible is attained before deciding to progress to an appliance for a patient. An appliance will control and often improve conditions which would otherwise have been regarded as chronic; where the patient would have had to pay regular visits to the surgery at intervals of, say, four weeks for the rest of his or her life, the use of a carefully designed appliance can mean that the treatments need be carried out less and less frequently. This could mean a reduction in income to the chiropodist, but in fact it has the opposite effect due to the raising of his professional reputation through the social contacts of his patients, and a far greater personal satisfaction in being able to do so much more for those who would otherwise have had to endure permanent disability to a greater or lesser degree.

Due attention must always be paid to the case history when assessing a condition for an appliance. What kind of padding and strapping has been used effectively in the past? How far can the condition be expected to improve with these methods? Has any fresh approach been neglected? If it is decided that the padding used has been as effective as it is reasonable to expect, if the condition appears to have improved as far as it can and no fresh approach in conventional materials seems likely to gain further ground, the answers to other questions must be sought. Are the shoes as suitable to the defect as the patient is likely to wear? Is the hosiery adequate? If an appliance which may be removed from the foot is envisaged, is the patient supple enough to reach the feet to perform this simple task? Has the patient the intelligence to use and treat the appliance with due regard to its advantages and limitations?

The shoe question is often a vexed one. The most universally suitable shoe for prolonged weight-bearing is accepted as being the lace-up type; due to the grip of properly placed laces, the shoe is held on the foot in such a way as to admit adequate function without excessive pressure or friction, especially in the area of the toes. In a properly fitting shoe of this type, the foot is unable to slide forward to allow the distal ends of the toes to meet the toe-box—this would cause back pressure on the toes, and through them the metatarsals, with resultant lesions and deformities. Thus any attempt to treat these lesions or deformities would meet with failure unless attention was paid to first causes. To fit an appliance designed to correct a foot in an environment which was achieving the opposite effect would be worse than useless. One or the other —the foot or the shoe—would give way in the end. At the same time, it would be unreasonable to expect, for instance, a professional ballet dancer or model to wear lace-up shoes, so there are occasions when compromise solutions must be found. This question will be discussed more fully later.

Hosiery should be long enough in the leg and foot to permit free movement. A stocking which is of sufficient length in the foot but too short in the leg will tend to 'ride up' at the heel, being then effectively too short in the foot. The 'stretch' type of stocking with its vague classification as to size, tends to limit free movement of the foot and should usually be discouraged; other problems are presented with this type of hosiery, but these would be irrelevant here.

When thinking of using a removable appliance for an elderly or disabled person, it is essential to ascertain not only that they can reach the foot comfortably but also that they are capable of putting the appliance in the right position. Apart from the more obvious complaints, such as those resulting in limitation of movement at the hip or knee, there are contra-indications to stooping (such as high blood pressure), near-sightedness where the patient perhaps also wears spectacles which have a fixed focal length, severe rheumatoid arthritis of the hands and so on. These, and others of the ills to which the flesh is heir, must all be taken into account if they are likely to restrict the activity of the patient sufficiently to affect their ability to cope with an appliance which depends for its success on accurate location relative to the condition it was designed to alleviate. There are ways of circumventing these objections which will be discussed in a later chapter, but a test of the efficiency of an appliance is the extent to which it is controlling and improving the condition for which it is designed, and not as is often erroneously assumed, the amount of comfort it gives.

The patient who has not the intelligence to wash the appliance occasionally or the wit to wear it on the correct foot, the right way up, in the right place and at the right time may seem to pose an unanswerable problem to the appliance maker. For example, a heavy manual labourer had been fitted with a 'glove' of latex with appropriate padding built into it and was given instructions as to its use and maintenance, being asked to return in two months for his next treatment. At the next visit he hobbled in, complaining that he had never been so uncomfortable, but when he removed his sock the ensuing stench prompted the question, 'When did you last take the appliance off?' This brought the answer, 'I've not had it off since it was put on for me last time.' The unwashed foot and appliance were very evident confirmation of the statement. 'Why not? Weren't you told to take it off each night, wash and dry it and your foot, and put it on again in the morning after powdering it?' A hurt, defensive look, then, 'Yes, but I was told I must wear it to work always.' 'Well?' 'But can't you see, I work night shifts!' Had he been told what to do when 'going to bed' and 'getting up' rather than 'at night' and 'in the morning', this unfortunate man would have been saved much unnecessary misery through an almost unbelievable misunderstanding. Any appliance should be clearly labelled as to which foot it is intended to fit, which side towards the skin and which way up; an indelible mark may be made on the appliance to indicate proximity to a permanent feature of the foot (such as a bony prominence) where this is plainly visible to the patient, remembering that the subtleties of surface marking so familiar to us are no more than mysteries to the patient.

The process of making the appliance is one which requires much care and which initially is very time consuming. As skill is acquired in the various techniques, so the amount of time spent begins to assume manageable proportions, but the construction of the properly finished and accurately fitting article should not be approached as a haphazard five minutes here, five minutes there affair. A well-run practice is a smoothly busy, well organised one. Somewhere it is necessary to fit in time for appliance work and time is a commodity of marketable value. To rely on the occasional cancellation of, or failure to keep an appointment to provide the requisite opportunity to, as it were, 'Throw something together for Mrs. Jones who's going on holiday next week', will usually result in something which will fail to satisfy aesthetic appearance, technical demand, or Mrs. Jones. Apart from these occasional and unreliable half-hour respites, or during the notorious seasonal slack periods of the practice, there are no opportunities to indulge in appliance work of any consequence and yet, if the modern chiropodist is to give a service of the scope which is reasonably expected today, such work is essential. The position appears to present an impasse. Thus a whole day or a large part of a working day should be set aside at regular intervals; appliance work will accumulate in the intervening time until there is sufficient to employ the reserved time profitably. Work can then be organised and spread out in its various stages without fear of interruption, and the cost of the time spent will be passed on to the patient in the fee for the appliance, thus satisfying all demands.

CHAPTER II

BASE, COVER, PADDING MATERIALS AND ADHESIVES

BASE MATERIALS

BASE materials, in the sense in which they are dealt with here, serve the purpose of providing a platform or basic shape on which to build an appliance to fit the foot, and which will fit in the shoe. There is quite a selection of materials from which to choose, ranging from cork, through various compounds to leather or sponge rubber, the choice depending upon different factors. There are three types which are most commonly used:

Regenerated Leather (or fibreboard). This consists of leather torn up into shreds and then bonded together with resin into sheets of even texture and thickness, the most useful thickness being either 1 mm. or 2 mm. The material is easily cut with scissors into differing shapes, and will withstand a fair amount of wear.

Cork Filled Rubber Sheeting. This consists of granulated cork bonded with rubber to give a sheet of the thickness desired of firm, though very flexible material which has the additional property of a mild degree of resilience. Due to the rubber content, this material resists slipping in the shoe.

Split Sponge Rubber. When this is used as a base material, $\frac{1}{16}$ in. in thickness is found to be most convenient. This material is of closed cell construction (the significance of which will be discussed later) and is very flexible.

COVER MATERIALS

In one form or another, leather is used for covering appliances. It is obtained by converting the hide of an animal into leather by the process known as 'Tanning', the details of which are not especially relevant here. Leather may be coloured by dyeing.

Skins vary according to the species from which they are taken, and also from animal to animal. They vary in texture, but are useful in this work for their properties of thickness and softness,

17

flexibility, 'elasticity' and their more or less neutral effect on the foot—which has become accustomed to a leather shoe.

Leather has a top surface, or 'grain' side, and an under surface, or 'flesh' side. The grain side is comparatively smooth and may be polished, when it will acquire a higher degree of moisture- and friction-resistance. The flesh side is found to be soft and 'furry'. The overall thickness of the material (and its strength) depends upon both the animal and the part of the animal from which it originates. Thus cow hide is thick and not very flexible if compared with glacé kid, persian lamb is much smoother than crocodile skin, and so on. When the 'flesh' is stripped off the 'grain' the result is two pieces of material, one (the top surface) being called 'skiver' leather, the other (the flesh side) being known as 'suède split'. Thus it is possible to obtain:

1. The complete skin, with grain and flesh sides not separated.
2. The grain side alone, as skiver leather, which may be bought up to a full skin size.
3. The flesh side alone, as suède split, again up to a full skin size.

These three basic types will be discussed in fuller detail under the heading of the appropriate skins.

There is a wide variety of choice of leathers in appliance work, but it will be found both economically and administratively expedient to use only four or five different kinds, of which the following are examples of some which have excellent differing qualities and uses:

1. Complete Skins

(a) *Persian Lamb*. This is a comparatively expensive leather, even though it does not come from any exotic breed of lamb in Persia. Its grain side feels smooth and soft to the touch and is capable of taking on quite a high polish. Its thickness and quality varies throughout the skin, as does that of any natural material, and it carries sufficient flesh to present difficulty in turning sharp corners. This difficulty may be surmounted in a manner to be described later.

(b) *French Basil*. Slightly heavier than persian lamb, this skin is not as flexible, but is useful for the student or beginner who needs practise in techniques which will eventually be applied to more expensive materials. Its grain side is a little coarser than that of persian lamb, although it will readily accept polish. The flesh side also is coarser, and it presents the same difficulty when required to turn sharp corners due to the grain side stretching over the crinkled flesh.

(c) *Glacé Kid*. A much lighter material than the foregoing examples, glacé kid has a particularly smooth or 'silky' grain surface and less thickness of flesh. This is one of the more expensive cover materials and gives a very good finished appearance, even without polishing.

2. Skiver Leather

As has already been indicated, skiver leather consists of the grain surface split away from the flesh, thus it is possible to buy up to a whole skin of skiver leather. Colour, as with other leathers, is no indication of quality, but merely shows that the material has been dyed. Since the flesh has been removed from skiver leather, it is very thin but still retains many of the characteristics of the original skin in so far that it will stretch in certain directions (depending upon which part of the skin it comes from), is fairly soft and will take polish.

3. Split Suède

This is the flesh side which has been stripped from the grain side of the leather. It might be described as 'furry' on both surfaces and before having further treatment it is uneven in thickness and texture. Split suède may be processed in a number of ways to yield differing results, two of which are amongst those useful in appliance work.

(a) *Chamois leather*. Although skins from sheep have so far formed the main basis for discussion, chamois is the flesh of leather of goat-antelope ancestry. Skins may be selected to be of fairly even consistency, but as it is an oil-dressed preparation, and the oil will not agree with either rubber padding or rubber adhesives, care should be exercised in the use to which this material is put. In practice, chamois leather will be found to become messy or 'goo-ey' after a time if used in conjunction with these materials.

(b) *Gas Meter Skin* (*Diaphragm leather*). This is a split suède which has been machined during its preparation to the even thickness to be used in the manufacture of the bellows in domestic and other gas meters. It may be obtained either as whole skins or as off-cuts known as 'Gas Meter Roundings' which will be found to be very cheap, although the time spent in sorting out suitable roundings tends to raise the cost again. Since this material has no oil dressing, its even thickness makes it a very suitable material for appliance work.

Artificial Cover Material

Thin sheets of regenerated leather bonded with rubber are obtainable, and these may be used for very simple insoles which have no complex contours (since the material does not take kindly to stretching). When compared with leather, the artificial material is cheap and has the great advantage that a more rapidly drying cement may be used on it than on the natural materials.

PADDING MATERIALS

The materials used in the construction of padding for incorporation in appliances differ from most, though not all, of those used in the surgery because there is need for them to perform their function for a much longer period than that expected of the day-to-day materials. Appliance padding materials must also be easy to use in conjunction with leathers, cork, cellulose acetate and rubber cements and so on. Accordingly, sponge rubbers are employed.

Structurally, there are two types of sponge rubbers for this work. There are those referred to as 'Closed Cell' and those known as 'Open Cell' sponge rubber materials, and these two differ very widely from each other in both structure and function.

1. Closed Cell Sponge Rubber

This consists of a mass of rubber containing very many small isolated pockets of gas distributed more or less evenly throughout the material. (Fig. 1) When weight is placed upon closed cell material, the isolated bubbles or cells of gas will change their shape but not their gas content, so although the material will compress to a certain extent, the pockets of trapped gas will exert back pressure on the weight as well as on the walls of the cells. (Fig. 2) When the weight is removed, each pocket of gas (and so the material itself) will resume its former shape. The gas contained in the cells is an inert one to avoid oxidation of the rubber material.

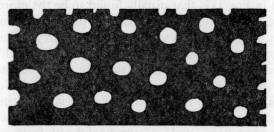

Fig. 1. Closed cell material, showing the skin side as a continuous line and the cell surface as a pitted line. Note that the bubbles of nitrogen are entirely separate from each other, being trapped in the rubber.

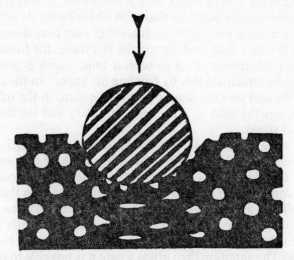

Fig. 2. A weight resting on closed cell material causes distortion of the underlying cells of gas with consequent redistribution of pressure and backthrust.

Nitrogen is often used for the purpose because, besides being inert, it is non-inflammable and also inexpensive.

Closed cell sponge rubber is obtainable either with both surfaces smooth (when it is referred to as skin/skin) or with one skin side and the other of cut cells, giving a rough surface; this last is called skin/cell, and is made by cutting skin/skin sponge rubber to half its original thickness. Since it gives a better finish to skive the material down to its skin surface and affords a smoother contour to start from the cell side, the skin/cell variety

(as shown in Fig. 1) is that usually found to be the more convenient. Closed cell material is supplied in thicknesses from $\frac{1}{16}$ in.,
$\frac{1}{8}$ in., $\frac{1}{4}$ in. and so on. To avoid wastage in carrying large stocks
of thick materials (which would be rarely used and would degener-
ate by oxidation during prolonged storage), it will be found useful
to store only those thicknesses already mentioned, building them
upon each other when needing thicker material as required, since
this will not in any way affect the function of the material.

Mention has been made of the backthrust from closed cell
material on weight bearing. The force of the backthrust on the
walls of the cells is equal to that of the weight placed upon it as
long as the ground or insole of the shoe gives solid resistance
underneath. If a man walks into a lamp-post, it will resist him
with a force exactly equal to that with which he hit it; action and
reaction are equal and opposite. If another man runs down a flight
of stairs two at a time and jumps the last three, the force hitting
his metatarsal area is equal to several tons, which is partly why
he is wise to anticipate this by bending his knees. In the one case
it could be said that the lamp-post hits the man, in the other that
the floor hits the man as if he were stationary and the floor were
moving at speed.

Now since closed cell material is capable of exerting quite
considerable backthrust whilst absorbing some of this on its cell
walls, it follows that it can be used for protection, for correction
or for a combination of both. It has already been seen that before
any appliance is made for a patient, treatments will have been
carried out using conventional padding materials (such as felt),
and as much result as could be reasonably expected will have been
achieved. The situation then arises where it is possible to translate
this padding into an appliance. If the intention behind the padding
hitherto used has been to correct something, adhesive felt, probably
semi-compressed, will have been used. The equivalent material
for felt is closed cell sponge rubber, and it will be found that since
felt tends to flatten during normal wear whereas closed cell
sponge rubber does not (to anything like the same degree), then
$\frac{1}{8}$ in. closed cell sponge rubber may be used in substitution for $\frac{3}{16}$ in.
felt, $\frac{1}{4}$ in. for $\frac{5}{16}$ in., $\frac{1}{2}$ in. for $\frac{5}{8}$ in. felt and so on.

2. Open Cell Sponge Rubber

(a) *Latex foam.* This consists of a mass of rubber honeycombed
with *interconnected* cells all of which, by means of each other,

communicate at the surfaces of the material with the atmosphere. (Fig. 3) Thus all the cells are filled with air at or near the temperature and humidity prevailing in the atmosphere in the immediate proximity. When weight is placed upon unsealed open cell material, it collapses instantly, leaving only the thickness of its rubber content between the weight and the structure supporting the material. (Fig. 4) When the weight is removed, the cells spring back to their usual shape and the material resumes its former dimensions.

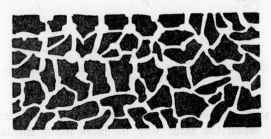

Fig. 3. Open cell material, showing how each cell is inter-connected with its neighbour and with the atmosphere.

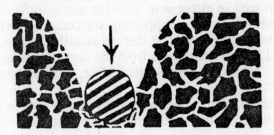

Fig. 4. A weight resting on open cell material causes the underlying material to be squashed flat while the rest is unaffected.

Since open cell material is made in such a way that all the cells can communicate through each other with the atmosphere outside the material it never has a 'skin' side, but it is possible to seal off all the surface cells from the outside air by covering the material completely with an airtight cover. The enclosed material will then behave as though it were an air cushion or single cell of air, and it can be used as a cushioning material. (Fig. 5)

Like closed cell sponge rubber, latex foam is supplied in varying thicknesses and can be obtained with an adhesive backing for use directly on the foot.

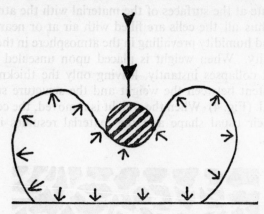

Fig. 5. The mode of behaviour of enclosed open cell material when a weight is placed upon it.

(b) *Polyurethane Foam.* This is another open cell material which behaves in much the same way as latex foam, although since it is made of a very light plastic—polyurethane—it has less 'body' in it, with the result that when it is not enclosed a weight will flatten it to such an extent as to leave the merest wafer of polyurethane between it and the supporting surface. Polyurethane has the advantage of being a good thermal insulator, and is therefore very useful in protecting areas from the heat caused by excessive friction, by taking the heat on its surface, so insulating the skin from its effect.

Polyurethane foam is used more in the surgery than in appliance work, due largely to the fact that rubber cements, being so versatile, are usually employed in this work and they work best with rubber material for padding. It is supplied either with or without adhesive backing in thicknesses of $\frac{1}{16}$ in., $\frac{3}{16}$ in., $\frac{5}{16}$ in., and so on, and may also be obtained in various tubular forms of differing thicknesses and sizes, with or without linings of one material or another, the object being to slip lengths of these over the toes.

ADHESIVES

Since most of the padding used in elementary appliance work is made of rubber, and the material which sticks best to rubber *is* rubber, the two basic adhesives which will be found to be of greatest use at this stage are rubber solution and latex rubber.

1. Rubber Solution. There are numerous types of rubber solutions on the market, the one most widely useful in appliance work being a solution of rubber in carbon tetrachloride (since this is free of sulphur or other impurities). In order to achieve good and complete adhesion between two rubber surfaces, it is only necessary to see that both are completely clean; thus it would be possible to stick together two pieces of rubber which had been scrupulously cleaned with a suitable solvent (such as carbon tetrachloride, for instance) were it not for the fact that some of the rubber on the surface of each will have become oxidised through contact with the air. To surmount this difficulty, rubber solution is used to clean both surfaces (thus adding some fresh rubber to the surfaces as well as cleaning them), but it is important to remember that the object of the exercise is to *clean* the surfaces, which should be rubbed vigorously to deposit only a thin layer of fresh rubber. Spreading rubber solution generously like marmalade will only take longer to dry and may result in slippage between the two layers of material. When the two prepared rubber surfaces are dry, they are pressed firmly together and may be hammered with a round-headed wooden mallet to establish good adhesion.

When using rubber solution, the lid of the tin should be kept in place as much as possible, as otherwise the carbon tetrachloride will evaporate, providing an unhealthy and unpleasant working atmosphere and also concentrating the remaining rubber solution into a thick, syrupy mass which may only be reconstituted after the addition of more solvent.

2. Latex Rubber. The use of rubber solution as an adhesive on leather involves two coats, the first being well hammered after it has dried and before applying the second, and even then the bond will not be the best attainable. The answer is to achieve a layer or skin of rubber on the flesh side of the leather (or on any porous non-rubber material) by coating it once evenly with latex, which sets or 'gels' across the peaks or roughnesses of the porous material whilst at the same time being firmly anchored to the surface by having permeated it to a certain extent before setting. The result is a good adhesion by providing a surface of clean rubber whilst retaining the flexibility of the material.

Latex rubber is not a rubber solution. It is the sap of the rubber tree, and contains between 30 per cent and 40 per cent natural rubber; this can be concentrated up to 75 per cent as required.

On exposure to air, the rubber coagulates rapidly because of evaporation of the moisture, but the rate of coagulation may be reduced by the introduction of an alkaline stabilising agent such as liquid ammonia, and it is this form which is used as an adhesive in appliance work.

Latex must be kept in a tightly sealed container, where it will keep in good condition for some months. It is better to keep a little latex taking up most of the space in a small container, in order not to trap more air in with the liquid than is strictly necessary, and during use the lid of the container should be lifted only for the time required, replacing it firmly between operations to prevent evaporation of the stabiliser with resultant coagulation of the rubber. Again, it is advisable to wear protective clothing whilst doing appliance work—a little latex spilt on any fabric will result in more than a stain, the area of fabric affected will have become rubberised.

A paint brush will be found to be very convenient for applying latex on to a surface as a thin coating, but it must be kept quite clean if all the bristles are not to set in a solid lump of rubber. The procedure is simple if always observed; first the brush is filled with soap solution and after squeezing out the excess soap it is dipped in latex, used as required and *before laying it down* it is washed out thoroughly under cold running water, dipped in the soap solution again, the excess solution squeezed out and if the brush will not be required again for some time it may then be washed out again under the cold running water.

Rubber solution, then, is rubber in solution in a solvent. If some of the solvent evaporates, more may be added, care being taken not to use too much and thin out the solution. The most convenient applicator for rubber solution is a small piece of waste closed cell sponge rubber, which, after repeated use will become very soft and unpleasant to handle due to the solvent dissolving some of the sponger rubber and making it tacky. The piece may then be discarded and a new one substituted.

Latex is rubber in *suspension*. To add more stabilising agent to latex which has been left open to the air will have little effect on the coagulated rubber. Care must be taken to wear protective clothing when using latex, which is applied to surfaces with a brush which must be kept quite clean. Latex takes some time to dry, for the water in the ammonia has to evaporate, leaving the once milky-looking latex to appear transparent. The drying process for latex may be speeded up by placing the work in a drying cabinet (at a temperature of about 65–70 deg. F.).

Although air may be circulated over work to be dried by using an electric fan, adhesives should *never* be dried by blowing on them, since moisture droplets in the breath will condense on the rubber surface and spoil proper adhesion.

CHAPTER III

SOME PRINCIPLES INVOLVED IN THE CHOICE OF PADDING MATERIALS

CHIROPODY as we know it today has a much greater scope than in the comparatively recent past. More can be done to help the patient in a number of ways than was the case only a few years ago; for instance, a wider range of padding materials is now available—materials which can act or can be made to act to counter the different kinds of irritating factors which produce lesions on the feet. To comprehend fully the forces acting in or on the foot, and to understand the capabilities of the materials to hand is to render a better service to the foot sufferer.

In the main, the force operating on the foot is friction, which may be one of two types: static or dynamic.

Static Friction

Static friction opposes an applied force. Suppose a tea-chest, too heavy to lift, is to be moved a few yards. It is pushed. At first quite a considerable force must be used to get it to move; the resistance to the thrust before the chest begins to move is the static friction between the base of the chest and the ground, and the greater the thrust, the higher the value of the static friction until the stage where the chest moves, when the static friction is overcome. Pushing now becomes easier, as dynamic friction is now occurring between the base of the chest and the ground and dynamic friction is of lower value than static, and heat is generated at the surfaces.

Another example: A weight resting upon a table exerts a certain known force upon the table and is resisted by an exactly equal and opposite force, action and reaction being equal and opposite. If the table is tilted slightly, the direction of thrust of the weight upon the table is altered, and the thrust is opposed by static friction (Fig. 6), the two forces being steadily greater in value until the weight begins to move, when the force of static friction ceases to exist; the point at which this happens depends upon the surfaces involved.

28

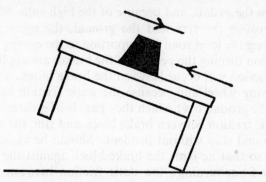

Fig. 6. An unmoving weight on an inclined surface does not slide off because of the equal and opposite resistance offered by static friction between the base of the weight and the surface with which it is in contact.

Dynamic Friction

Dynamic friction is the resistance offered to an applied force between moving surfaces. The tea-chest, in the first example, was pushed hard enough to begin to slide. The resistance offered to the movement between the sliding surfaces of the base of the chest and the ground is dynamic friction which, though of lower value than static friction, produces heat (here being produced by work as a force operating through a distance). In the second example, when the table was tilted to a sufficient degree to overcome the static friction between the weight and the table-top, there was dynamic friction between the moving surfaces and heat was generated. A man walks along a pavement. Each part of the sole of his shoe, in relation to each part of the pavement upon which he walks, is stationary, unmoving, so his muscles and momentum push against the static friction between the sole of his shoe and the ground, and he progresses in the opposite direction to that in which he pushes. He begins to hurry, pushing harder against the static friction, and (as long as he does not slip) he runs; suddenly someone walks across his path and he tries to stop his feet from moving on the pavement, but the force of his momentum is such as to overcome the static friction (of high value) between the soles of his shoes and the ground so that his shoes will slide along the ground (lower value dynamic friction), generating heat, wearing away his shoe-leather and causing him to fall. Another example: Each part of the tyre of a bicycle wheel, in relation to the corresponding part of the road surface, is stationary as the cyclist turns the pedals, and because of the high value of the static friction between the tyre and the ground, the cycle progresses steadily along the level road in proportion to the energy the cyclist expends upon turning the pedals. If the brakes are applied gently, dynamic friction will occur between the brake blocks and the rim of the moving wheel and because the static friction between the tyres and the ground over which they pass is of greater value than the dynamic friction between brake block and rim, the cyclist will slow down and stop without incident. Should he violently apply his brakes so that he jams the brake block against the wheel (so stopping it from turning), the static friction between the brake block and wheel will be of such a high value as to keep the wheel locked and drag the tyre along the surface of the road, opposed only by dynamic friction, giving a skid, possible loss of control and heating up the tyre so that some of its substance will be left on the road surface.

The heat produced by dynamic friction can burn the tissues of the body. Outstanding examples of this can be found in sliding down a rope (whilst not gripping tightly enough to climb down) or in a fall, being flung across the surface of the ground. In either event, burns will be caused to the tissues, altering their chemistry. In a similar manner, though to a much lesser degree, the heat generated by dynamic friction (e.g. between a loose shoe and the foot) unless dispersed rapidly by conduction through the underlying soft tissues, can alter the chemistry of the skin cells when allied with shearing stress in such a way that scaling may occur, building up layer upon layer to form callous. Thus a chemical change will result from a physical force.

So, when standing still, the force of static friction, combined with compressive stress, is brought to bear on the skin of the foot. When walking, especially in a loose shoe, dynamic friction occurs with shearing stress, generating heat on the skin which, if unprotected by the underlying superficial fascia, will alter the chemistry of the skin cells to form callous. Thus the body tissues are almost constantly under stress of one kind or another, and there is a system of measurement of the behaviour of material when it is exposed to stress, called Moduli.

Moduli

There are three kinds of moduli of interest in chiropody (since this is a field concerned only with certain kinds of stress).

1. *The modulus of Elasticity* (*Mod. E.*). This is a measurement of the power within a material to resist change of length, and of the ability of the material to return to its original length (in the manner of a pulled or pushed rod; pull or push with sufficient force and it will eventually change its length, release it and measure to see if it has returned to its original length). The Mod. E. could be said to be a measurement of the power within a material to resist *stretching* or elongation. For instance, if a strong force meets with little resistance (to stretching or pushing), the resistance is expressed as having a low Mod. E. On the other hand, if a steel ball is dropped on to a sheet of plate glass it will bounce high, because both the ball and the glass have a high Mod. E., whereas if a rubber ball is dropped on to a sheet of rubber, it will hardly bounce at all as rubber has a low Mod. E.

2. *The modulus of Bulk or Compression* (*Mod. K.*). This is a measurement of the power within a material to resist *squeezing* or change of size in the sense of volume when under uniform stress over its whole surface. For example, a liquid will strongly resist attempts to change its volume (it is upon this principle that hydraulic pumps work), and so has a high Mod. K.

3. *The modulus of Rigidity* (*Mod. n.*). As the name implies, this is a measurement of the power within a material to resist *crushing* or change of shape.

Stress

Where appliance work is concerned, in the main there are two types of stress, although a third is a combination of the two. These are (1) *Tensile stress*, (2) *Compressive stress*, and the combination of both is called (3) *Shear*.

1. *Tensile stress* is the reaction within a material to attempts at changing its length. If a cube of material were to have a force applied to it pushing in one direction on its upper surface and resisted by an equal opposite force on its lower surface (Fig. 7), the reaction in cross-section parallel to the two opposite corners C B is that of tensile stress. Another form of stress would be set up in the same cube subjected to this treatment. . . .

2. *Compressive stress* is the reaction within a material to attempts at changing its size (in the sense of volume). Thus, in the example, compressive stress would be set up perpendicularly between AB and CD (Fig. 8) as well as diagonally parallel to AD. . . .

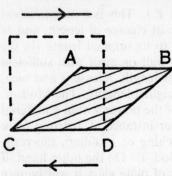

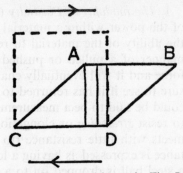

Fig. 7. The dotted lines indicate the original shape of the cube, the arrows show the direction of the applied forces. The stripes parallel to CB show where tensile stress is set up.

Fig. 8. The same cube as in Fig. 7, subjected to the same applied forces, will show compressive stress between AB and CD.

3. So two types of stress are set up in the same cube which, taken together, constitute *shearing stress*. A cylinder, subjected to opposing forces twisting it, is subjected to radial shear, torque or torsion. (Fig. 9)

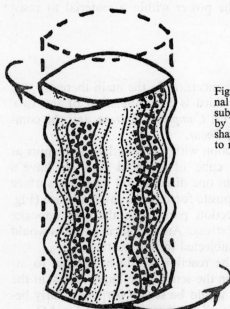

Fig. 9. The dotted lines show the original shape of the cylinder which, when subjected to opposing forces as shown by the arrows, twists to assume this shape. The cylinder has been subjected to radial shear.

Now solids tend to resist both tensile and compressive stress, exhibiting high Mods. E., K., and n. The more 'solid' the solid, the higher the modulus.

Liquids offer high resistance to squeezing, but very little to stretching or crushing, showing a high Mod. K., but low Mods. E. and n.

Gases offer virtually no resistance to change of length, volume or shape, showing low Mods. E., K., and n.

Insulation and Protection

How is this outline study of the physics of friction, stress and strain related to chiropody and appliance work?

Friction, whether static or dynamic, occurs all over the body (between bones at joints, between muscles and other soft tissues, and between skin and the surfaces with which it comes into contact) which normally has its own defence mechanism to afford protection from any harmful effects. At joints there are special articular surfaces and the presence of synovial fluid to act as lubrication. Individual muscles are surrounded by a connective tissue sheath which is called the epimysium, between tendon and retinacula or adjacent soft tissues there are tendon sheaths, and beneath the skin (especially at weight-bearing points) there is the thickness of the superficial fascia. The superficial fascia helps to protect the underlying tissues from:

1. Heat or cold.
2. Pressure.

1. The thermal insulation provided by the superficial fascia is afforded partly by the action of the sweat glands in the skin, and partly by the globules of fat which, being poor conductors of heat, are good insulators both against external heat and external cold. This is important in many ways, but in this context it protects from the heat generated by dynamic friction on the skin.

2. The protection from pressure (in the form of compressive and shearing stress) is in the main afforded by the superficial fascia. The liquid fat has, of course, a high modulus of compression, resisting squeezing, and since each globule is enclosed, if localised compressive stress falls on a small area of skin, it is dispersed or redistributed before it reaches the underlying bone; pressure is a force on unit area, the area of skin was small, but by the time the force reaches the bone it has been spread out by the superficial

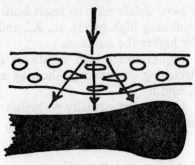

Fig. 10. Pressure falling on a small area of the skin is spread out by the closed cell nature of the globules of fat so that it falls on a wider area of the soft tissues between it and the bone.

fascia and the area has become correspondingly larger. (Fig. 10)

In chiropody, materials are used which have various different properties. All are designed to give protection; some give protection from compressive stress by redistributing it over the skin surface (in cases where there is diminution of the superficial fascia, cushioning materials are used), some by redistribution in such a way that the materials themselves take the pressure over a wider area (corrective materials), and some can be made to give thermal insulation alone. All, then, are protective, but in the words of a famous broadcaster, 'It depends on what you mean by the word' protective.

Some examples of materials in common use in relation to their properties are:

MATERIAL	MADE OF	PROPERTY
Z.O. Strapping	Cotton and rubber	Takes some of the heat from dynamic friction on its surface.
Stockinette	Looser texture cotton and rubber	Takes more heat than strapping on its surface due to the trapped air within its looser texture, though its main value lies in its one-way stretch.
Fleecy Web	Stockinette with the 'nap' of the cotton raised	Holds more air than stockinette initially, but retains more moisture (a good conductor of heat). As it wears, it reverts to stockinette.

MATERIAL	MADE OF	PROPERTY
Wool Felt	A mass of wool, with air interspersed. Spread with Z.O. adhesive	Also compresses and fills with moisture, holding more than stockinette or fleecy web, so it loses its thermal insulation. Wool felt will not respond very readily to movement of the skin and is used for corrective padding rather than for cushioning or thermal insulation.
Latex Foam	Rubber, with inter-connected air pockets in its mass, to give open cell sponge rubber. (Fig. 3)	Due to its construction, this material is used wholly for cushioning, though to be effective in this way, the whole of its surface must be made airtight so that pressure upon it cannot make the air within escape. (Fig. 5)

Polyurethane Foam This is made from crude oil, which is heated to produce—

CRUDE OIL   plus   HEAT   with   CATALYST

↓

AROMATICS   HEAVY FRACTIONS   CRACKER GAS

The cracker gas was regarded as a waste by-product, and since it is a highly toxic gas, it used to be burned off. Today, however, its components are utilised by synthesis into polymers, the basis of the plastics industry—

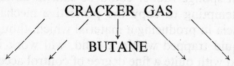

CRACKER GAS

BUTANE

METHANE ETHANE   PROPANE URETHANE

↓

POLYURETHANE (by polymerisation)

Polyurethane foam is familiar today as draught excluding material, lagging material and in many spheres where insulation is required. In chiropody, it is probably the most efficient insulating material available at the present time. It will withstand heat up to 100 deg. C., and if a limb is covered with polyurethane foam and some poly-vinyl-chloride ('P.V.C.') is heated to a high temperature, when it becomes mouldable, the hot P.V.C. may be placed on to the polyurethane-covered limb, because the polyurethane will not give up the heat from the P.V.C. as it is such a poor conductor. Thus, when the skin is subjected to dynamic friction, and the heat generated cannot be dispersed by reason of an inadequate superficial fascia, polyurethane foam may be placed on it and the dynamic friction will then occur on the surface of the foam, which will insulate the heat from the underlying skin which is then subjected only to static friction (from which there is no heat).

Thus, polyurethane foam is an open cell material which is an outstandingly good insulator. Latex foam is also of open cell construction, is not such a good insulator, but if covered with an airtight cover will act as a cushion or single large cell of air.

The characteristics of a material required to give correction are:

1. It must not easily change shape, so must have a high Mod. n.
2. It may often need to be flexible.

It has been shown that there are a number of materials which display the requisite characteristics, but in appliance work—where rubber is mainly used for padding and as adhesive—closed cell sponge rubber is the choice for corrective padding. This consists of columns of rubber interspersed with isolated pockets of inert gas. Solids resist pressure, but gas does so only by changing its shape and volume, so there are grades of closed cell sponge rubber which contain differing amounts of the inert gas; so, to use closed cell sponge rubber could be said to be learning from nature by attempting to copy the protective mechanism of the superficial fascia in producing a material which, though using gas instead of liquid trapped within a solid, will work in much the same way, and with quite a fine degree of control according to the choice of the grade of closed cell sponge rubber.

CHAPTER IV

NON-CASTING TECHNIQUES

PLANTAR metatarsal padding may take a variety of forms and positions on the plantar surface of the foot, these being governed by the function they are designed to fulfil. Accordingly, it is necessary to begin with a definition of terms.

A plantar metatarsal pad, when considered in relation to its full thickness or operative area, may be thought of as one in which the anterior edge conforms to the line of the 2nd, 3rd and 4th metatarso-phalangeal joints, the medial and lateral edges just into the 1st and 4th intermetatarsal spaces, and the posterior edge lies approximately two-thirds of the length towards the bases of the metatarsal shafts. (Fig. 11) Skiving, or bevelling, is of an equal depth to the thickness of the material used at the anterior, medial and lateral edges, and about twice this at the posterior edge; this is referred to as 'short' or 'normal' and 'long' skiving respectively (Figs. 12 and 13)

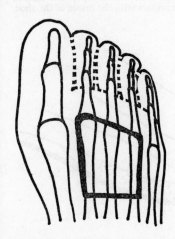

Fig. 11. The extent and position of the full thickness of a metatarsal pad in relation to the underlying bones on the plantar surface of the foot at rest.

When weight is first placed upon the foot with the pad in this position, the immediate effect is that the heads of the 2nd, 3rd and 4th metatarsals begin to yield to the increased pressure by being

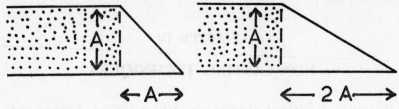

Fig. 12. 'Short' or 'Normal' skiving.   Fig. 13. 'Long' skiving.

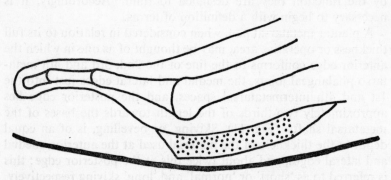

Fig. 14. A longitudinal cross-section through the second, third or fourth toe and its metatarsal with the metatarsal pad in position (the shaded area represents the full thickness of the pad). This is the moment before impact with the insole of the shoe.

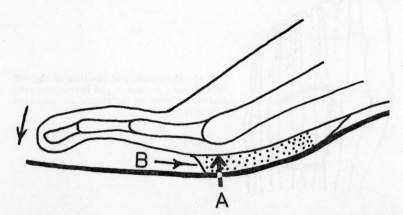

Fig. 15. The first moment of weight-bearing. The metatarsal head rises in response to pressure (A) from the full thickness of the pad, the apex of the toe is being brought into contact with the insole of the shoe, and a backwards traction (B) begins on the skin. Pressure is thus redistributed: (1) On to the toe, and (2) backwards along the shaft of the metatarsal.

raised, so bringing the toes down into firmer contact with the insole of the shoe. This effect on the toes is heightened by the backwards traction on the skin. (Figs. 14 and 15) In walking, the momentary raising of the metatarsal heads is not as important as the longer-lasting skin traction (Fig. 15); as the heel is raised, (Fig. 16) so the full thickness of the pad is carried behind those parts of the metatarsal heads which are now nearest to the insole of the shoe—until at the stage of final take-off the pad is having no effect at all. (Fig. 17) A metatarsal pad *relieves pressure* from

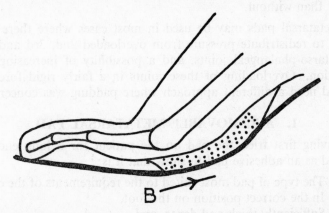

Fig. 16. As the heel is raised, the pad is being squeezed backwards (B) with more and more pressure, so maintaining and increasing toe action by skin traction.

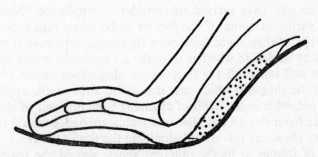

Fig. 17. The moment before take-off. The metatarsal pad has completed its cycle of activity, achieved its object, and ceased to function until the next step.

overloaded metatarso-phalangeal joints in the following ways:

1. A minimal effect. By raising the metatarsal heads, thus

altering the *time* at which they will come into play.

2. By creating a backwards pull or *traction* on the skin. As the heel is raised, this increases as the backthrust on the pad becomes more pronounced.

3. By *redistributing* the pressure in two directions:

   (i) Backwards along the metatarsal shafts,
   (ii) On to the toes.

Pressure is a force per unit area and the area presented to the insole of the shoe is greater with the pad in position than without.

Metatarsal pads may be used in most cases where there is a need to redistribute pressure from overloaded 2nd, 3rd and 4th metatarso-phalangeal joints, and a possibility of increasing toe function. Overloading of these joints in a fairly rigid forefoot would need a different approach where padding was concerned.

1.   A REMOVABLE METATARSAL PAD

Having first tried the pad on the patient for a long enough period as an adhesive pad to show that it is:

1. The type of pad most suited to the requirements of the case,
2. In the correct position on the foot,
3. Sufficiently thick and dense, and
4. That no further progress in treatment can be expected in the near future using this adhesive pad,

the time will have arrived to consider an appliance. Note was made earlier of some of the factors to be taken into account at this stage. When these have been thoroughly analysed it will be necessary to decide whether to make an appliance which may be put on and taken off the foot—something which *moves with the foot* in the shoe—in which case it is called a *removable* appliance. If the patient is in the habit of changing from one pair of shoes to another from day to day, the removable appliance would be the obvious choice as this would eliminate the need to make a whole series of insoles to fit the different shoes; should the patient be unable to reach the feet to place the appliance in the correct position, this type would be unsuitable.

The size, shape, position, density and thickness of the pad will have already been determined from the adhesive padding which had been used with optimum results. There are several methods in current use of translating this information into a removable appliance; some use a system of paper patterns, some the backing from the adhesive pad, some a duplicate pad and some a system of measurements recorded on a card. To discuss all the methods here would occupy too much space, each way has its merits (more than one road leads to London), but the one which gives a permanent record of the work carried out for the patient will be discussed here.

The measurement system*

Although the paper pattern and other methods have been in use for many years, in private practice it has been found that they have certain disadvantages, not the least of which was the absence of permanent records of the details of each appliance (which does not make sense when it is remembered with what care the competent chiropodist writes up the case and treatment notes on the patient's card). Situations would arise where the patient would lose his (perhaps new) appliance when on holiday, or would feel that it had been so successful that he would like an exact duplicate. It has even happened that one ex-patient, who had emigrated to South Africa some three years previously, wrote in (with the consent of his South African chiropodist) to ask for four pairs of appliances 'Exactly the same as last time' to be sent out to him. Although it is common knowledge that changes take place in the foot as the years go by, and as the appliance being worn has its effect—and the measurement system will keep a faithful record of this—the efficient chiropodist should be in a position to help his patient whenever such help is needed. Patterns or duplicate pads are difficult to store and identify in any quantity; frequently, receptionists charged with this duty fail to appreciate the enormity of the offence if they inadvertently mislay a marked length of strapping, a piece of paper, or a pad, whereas they more easily realise that record cards are not only important but also easy to file and maintain in alphabetical order. A filing cabinet full of cards is not only easier to keep in order, but also gives ease of access to information at short notice.

Bearing these considerations in mind, the author has devised and successfully operated for some years a method which overcomes these difficulties in several ways. Firstly, it takes 1 mm. as

*An outline on which this is based was first published in *The Chiropodist*, Vol. XVIII, 4, April 1963, page 113.

Appliance Record Card

Name............................. Case No...........

Address .... Tel:..............

....

Date	
Foot	Left
Met. Form	2>1>3>4>5
L.P.	65
W.P.	45>40
L.B.	180
W.B.	52
B.T. (mid.)	32
B.T. (lat.)	22
Loop M	35
Loop Lat.	10
L. Loop	120(8)
Materials and Notes	¼ in. c.c., elastic webbing, gas meter skin. O/c insert to loop; (30)60
Date Completed	

Fig. 18

the unit of measurement. This allows a similarly restricted margin of error which proves, in practice, to be as high a degree of accuracy as could be required, as well as dispensing with arithmetical problems over fractions of inches when the mind should be free to concentrate on the real nature of the job in hand. Secondly, it keeps a permanent record of all the relevant details of the appliance which may, at a later date, be of value in reproducing a duplicate, or in noting exactly any modifications to the original. All the measurements and notes are made on a card (Fig. 18) which bears the name, address and telephone number of the patient together with any other relevant information. These appliance measurement cards may either be kept in a separate file or attached to the treatment record cards, although the former is preferable since the treatment cards may be left in the file whilst the appliance card is in use. Thirdly, the method of measurement takes into account the mobile nature of the structure for which the appliance is designed, and makes exact allowances for this in so far as a correct diagnosis and evaluation of the case has been carried out.

The main principle underlying the method is that all measurements are taken either longitudinally or transversely—they are at right angles to each other—so they must bear relation to one fixed longitudinal and one fixed transverse line, as with the grid reference system in cartography. In applying this to the metatarsal pad on a metatarsal band, the *longitudinal line* is that of the *fourth intermetatarsal space* on the medial side of the 5th metatarsal, and the *transverse line* is that of the *leading edge of the metatarsal band* which is placed so that it runs from just behind the 5th metatarsal head across the plantar surface of the foot at right angles to the longitudinal line.

Measurement. A transparent ruler marked off in millimetres is the most suitable measuring device since this may be placed over, rather than adjacent to, the points of measurement, readings being taken through it so increasing the accuracy achieved. Before any figures are noted, the name and other details of the patient are recorded in the place provided at the top of the card, then, at the top of what will constitute a vertical list of measurements, appears the date. When measurements are taken for future appliances, these will appear on the right of their preceding measurements, each headed by the date on which they were taken, and on the following line a note 'right' or 'left', followed by the metatarsal formula for that foot (this is necessary at a later stage to determine the shape of the leading edge of the pad, which is, of course, directly linked to the relative positions of the metatarsal heads). The measurements will be those of the pad which is visualised as being already in place.

At first using this method, the foot—or the pad on the foot— may be marked with a ball-point pen, but subsequently the length of the pad is measured on the bare foot by placing the ruler parallel to the fourth intermetatarsal space, measuring from the anterior tip to the posterior edge at the longest part of the pad. (Fig. 19) A note of the reading is made so: L.P. 65 (length of pad, 65 mm.). Now the ruler is placed transversely over the metatarsal heads so that it lies at right angles to the line of the fourth inter-space, and a reading is taken of the distance between the most medial and the lateral edges of the pad (Fig. 19) with the ruler held in this position; this is an instance of the use of the trans-parency of the ruler through which readings are taken. A note of the measurement is made thus: W.P. 45 (width of pad, 45 mm.). A measurement of the pad at its posterior border is taken trans-versely from the lateral edge (Fig. 19) and noted alongside the previous measurement thus: W.P. 45>40.

The next measurement concerns the metatarsal band. A length of the material to be used in the actual appliance (in this case, elastic webbing) is placed around the forefoot so that its leading edge comes just behind the prominence of the 5th metatarsal head

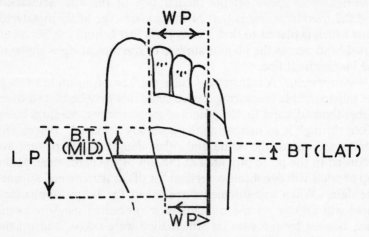

Fig. 19. Measuring a metatarsal pad.

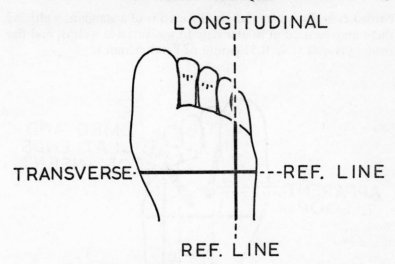

Fig. 20. The longitudinal reference line lies along the medial side of the 5th metatarsal, and the transverse line is at right angles to it (arising from just behind the head of the 5th metatarsal).

on the lateral border, and runs across the plantar surface at right angles to the 4th interspace. (Fig. 20) The required tension is applied to the elastic webbing as it is held in place, and the point at which the material overlaps its free end is marked with a ball-point pen, tension then being relaxed but the band being kept in position for two further measurements. The relative position of the pad to the band must be recorded in addition to another measurement which will be needed in arriving at the shape of the leading edge of the pad. So, measuring from the leading edge of the band (the transverse reference) to the *most anterior tip* of the pad in the longitudinal plane, (Fig. 19) a note of the reading is made: B.T. (mid.) 32 (band to anterior tip of pad in the region of the mid-line of the foot, 32 mm.). The second measurement is taken in the 4th intermetartarsal space from the anterior edge of the band to the anterior tip of the pad (Fig. 19) and noted thus: B.T. (lat.) 22 (band to anterior tip of pad at the longitudinal reference line, 22 mm.). The 'dummy' band is removed from the foot and a note made of the distance between the free end and the mark made when it was under the appropriate tension. This measurement is then noted: L.B. 180 (length of band unstretched, 180 mm.). The required width of the band is measured and recorded even if the material usually used is of a standard width, as there may be need at a later date to use variable widths, and the reading is noted: W.B.52 (width of band, 52mm.).

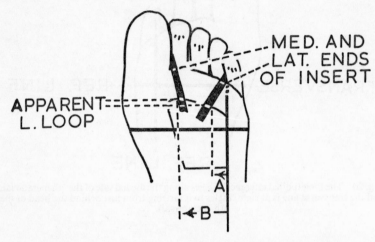

Fig. 21. A is the measurement 'Loop Lat.', B is that for 'Loop M'.

For the toe loop, a length of folded zinc oxide strapping is placed in position and marked at its points of intersection with the leading edge of the pad (the lateral mark being marked 'lateral') as well as at the ends of where the open cell 'insert' or cushioning pad will be. (Fig. 21) Before removing the 'dummy' loop, the distance between the medial side of the medial attachment and the longitudinal reference line ('B' in Fig. 21) is measured in the transverse plane and noted: Loop M, 35 (loop medial, 35 mm.). The distance between the lateral side of the lateral attachment and the longitudinal reference line is measured ('A' in Fig. 21) and recorded: Loop Lat. 10. Now the 'dummy' loop is removed and the distance between the marks appearing on it furthest apart is noted with the intended width of the loop in brackets: L. Loop 120 (8). Now the distance from the lateral mark to the lateral end of the open cell insert (30) is noted in brackets, followed by the distance between the two middle marks and both are noted under the heading 'Materials and Notes': O/c insert to loop (30) 60. (Fig. 18) Finally, a list is made of the materials used for the appliance, together with details as to thickness, skiving, and footnotes about any unusual features: this is followed by the date on which the appliance is completed.

The time taken in the surgery for marking and recording the measurements will not be more than two minutes once skill has been acquired in using the method. If the readings are dictated to a receptionist or to a tape recorder, there is an even greater economy in time. Apart from normal surgery equipment, all that is required for this stage is:

1. A length of elastic webbing (which may be used a number of times) for the metatarsal band.
2. A transparent plastic ruler, clearly marked in millimetres.
3. A supply of cards with the code letters printed or duplicated in the left-hand margin.
4. A ball-point pen.

The card now bears all the necessary information for the preparation of an appliance which will fit to a margin of error of 1 mm.

Translation of the Measurements. Where adhesives are concerned, the making of the appliance will occupy two stages, that involving latex, and that involving rubber solution. Since latex takes some time to dry, it is wise to prepare the latexed surfaces before commencing the rest of the procedure, thus avoiding holding the completion up during the final stages. Those surfaces which will be coated with latex are:

1. The cover material.
2. The loop attachments.
3. Part of the elastic webbing.

1. The amount of cover material may be calculated from the measurements by taking the B.T. (mid.) reading, adding to this the W.B. reading, and adding a further 5 mm. to give room for manoeuvre (32 plus 52 plus 5 equals 89 mm.); so the minimum length of each of the two pieces of gas meter skin required in this instance will be 89 mm. The minimum width of each piece of cover material is that of the pad at its widest, with an additional 2 or 3 mm. (45 plus 2 equals 47 mm.). So two rectangles, 89 mm. by 47 mm. marked with a ball-point pen on the gas meter skin, cut out, one side of each is coated with latex and then they are put to one side to dry.

2. The material required for the loop attachment is marked out on the gas meter skin by taking the 'apparent' L. loop measurement 120(8) ('A' in Fig. 22), marking off a strip at least 40 mm. longer than this (to allow for the anchoring tabs 'D' in Fig. 22) with the measurement in the centre, and making the width of the strip double the figure in brackets. In this instance, a strip at least 160 mm. long will be marked 20 mm. from each end and will be 16 mm. wide. Two further marks must appear on this strip, these representing the positions of the two ends of the open cell sponge insert; from the notes on the card, it will be seen that from a position 30 mm. from the lateral point of attachment, ('C' in Fig. 22) the insert extends 60 mm. towards the medial attachment. ('B' in Fig. 22) The strip is now cut from the material and coated with latex, being then laid aside to dry.

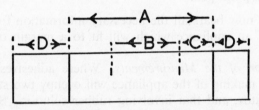

Fig. 22. The material for the toe loop marked out before coating with latex. Here: A represents the 'Apparent' length of the loop, B the length of the insert, C the lateral attachment to the co-ordinate for the commencement of the insert, and D is the material allowed for anchorage.

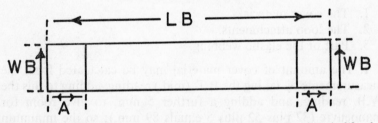

Fig. 23. The material for the metatarsal band cut out, with each end marked for the level of dipping in latex.

3. The two ends of the elastic webbing which are to attach to the appliance must be treated with latex. Elastic webbing is made of elastic—rubber—strands covered with cotton thread wound round and round each strand. These cotton threads are porous

and must be soaked with latex if they are to achieve good adhesion. So when the requisite amount of material (in this case, the length of the band was 180 mm.) has been cut from the roll, marks are made at each end at half the width of the pad at the transverse reference, to indicate the length of the webbing to be treated with latex. ('A' in Fig. 23) A method of ensuring that the cotton-covered material is fully covered with latex is to dip each end separately into the liquid up to the indicating mark (Fig. 24); as the webbing is withdrawn from the latex, it is pulled gently through or between the index and third fingers of the disengaged hand (Fig. 25), the material being then hung up to dry so that both its free ends are pendant. (Fig. 26)

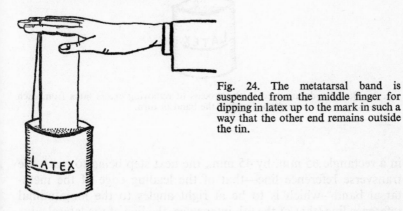

Fig. 24. The metatarsal band is suspended from the middle finger for dipping in latex up to the mark in such a way that the other end remains outside the tin.

All the materials to be treated with latex will now be in various stages of drying, and attention may be turned to the pad itself.

The Pad. The measurements on the card give the basic information needed to show the rectangle within the limits of which lies the pad (touching, or in two cases, conforming to its borders).

There is a note of the *length* of the pad at its longest under the heading L.P., 65 mm. in this case. All markings on the closed cell sponge rubber will be made on the skin side, since the skiving of the pad will be *away* from the foot so that the flat surface of the pad will be presented to the insole of the shoe (itself relatively flat). Thus the closed cell sponge rubber is placed flat on the work bench with its skin side uppermost, and two parallel lines are drawn on it 65 mm. apart. Taking the measurement between the most medial and the lateral borders of the pad (W.P. 45), two parallel lines at right angles to those already marked are drawn, resulting

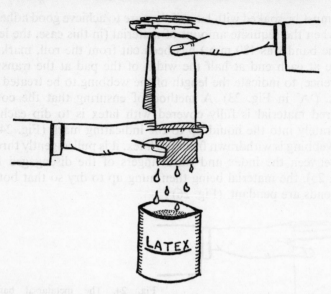

Fig. 25. Both hands are used in the process of removing excess latex from each dipped end of the band in turn.

in a rectangle 65 mm. by 45 mm., the next step being to mark the transverse reference line—that of the leading edge of the meta-tarsal band—which is to be at right angles to the longitudinal reference line (that of the 4th interspace, the line of the lateral edge of the pad). The transverse reference line is found by using the measurement B.T. (mid.)—here 32—and marking *both* edges of

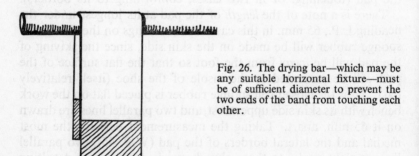

Fig. 26. The drying bar—which may be any suitable horizontal fixture—must be of sufficient diameter to prevent the two ends of the band from touching each other.

the rectangle 32 mm. from its anterior edge, joining the marks with a line which will be parallel to the anterior and posterior borders. (Fig. 27) The metatarsal formula shows that the second

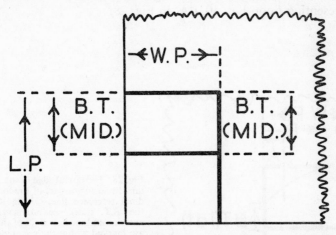

Fig. 27. The basic rectangle marked on the skin side of a sheet of closed cell sponge rubber. Note that the B.T. (mid.) measurement gives the transverse reference line which is parallel to the anterior edge of the rectangle.

metatarsal head lies anterior to the first, which in turn lies anterior to the third, which again is anterior to the fourth. In plotting the shape of the leading edge of the pad, then, there will evidently be a pronounced curve. The position of the second is already measured and marked (B.T. (mid.)), that of the fourth has been measured (B.T. (lat.)) but not yet marked, and the contour of the curve is known. Each of the middle three metatarsal heads will occupy approximately one-third of the width of the pad. Measuring forward along the lateral edge of the rectangle, the point 22 mm. from the transverse reference line is marked (B.T. (lat.) 22), and using the known facts already mentioned, the shape of the anterior edge of the pad is drawn in. (Fig. 28) The form of the medial edge of the pad is determined by using the measurement W.P. 45>40. Measuring along the posterior edge of the rectangle, the point 40 mm. from the longitudinal reference line is marked, and the shape is sketched in from there to the medial end of the border of the pad as already marked. Finally, the points for the loop attachments must be indicated. Taking 'Loop M.35', the point on the anterior edge of the pad which is 35 mm. transversely from the longitudinal reference line is marked ('B' in Fig. 28), and in the same way the point on the anterior edge of the pad which is 10 mm. from the longitudinal reference line (in this case the lateral edge of the rectangle)—measuring transversely—is marked, this representing Loop Lat. 10. ('A' in Fig. 28)

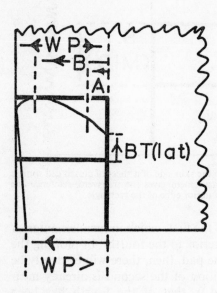

Fig. 28. The lateral edge of the meta-tarsal pad forms part of the longitudinal reference line. Using it and the B.T. (lat.) measurement, the anterior and medial edges of the pad are marked within the rectangle and the positions for the loop attachments marked at the anterior edge.

The pad is now fully marked out and ready to be cut from the sheet of closed cell sponge rubber as soon as the name of the patient has been marked on it.

Basic Principles. Whilst taking the measurements and translating them into the appliance, scrupulous care must be exercised to see that each reading is taken and recorded under its proper heading and that it is taken in no other direction than parallel to the reference lines. The basis of success with this system is not only its speed but also its reliability and accuracy, although it should be remembered that the measurements are those of the ideas of the operator as to shape, size and positioning of the appliance, basing these on work previously carried out in ordinary adhesive materials. Guesswork must be ruled out: one mistake or minor dishonesty with oneself in the early stages will upset all the calculations. Clear judgement, followed by accurate measurements, will give unfailingly first-class results. Discussion will follow, under the appropriate headings, on applying the measurement principle to single or double wing pads, cavity covers, 'U-ed' cover pads and so on, but it will have been seen that the basic principle of using one fixed longitudinal and one fixed transverse line in relation to the underlying structures may be applied to a wide variety of appliances the pad of which is intended to be relatively flat. Imagine a wire net of square 1 mm. mesh placed over the plantar surface of a foot with a pad in position. Two of the wires, one longitudinal and one transverse, are painted red, positioned at predetermined points, and serve as 'zero'. All measurements are taken using these as references. The beauty of the method lies in its ease of operation, its accuracy and reliability, and its provision of complete permanent records relating to each appliance with which the patient may, over the years, be provided.

Assembling the Appliance. First, the pad must be skived on the cell side in the usual way, thus leaving all markings on the skin side undisturbed. Next, the cell side of the pad is cleaned with rubber solution and placed skin side down on the bench to dry, a matter of two or three minutes. Here it is of interest to note that when sponge rubber has been cleaned with rubber solution, it buckles whilst the solution is still wet and resumes its normal shape when dry again (a useful guide as to when the surface is dry); this is due to the fact that the solvent in the rubber solution dissolves the surface to which it is applied as the fresh rubber which was in the solution is added to the surface, which consequently expands, settling down again as the solvent evaporates off.

When the cell side of the pad is dry, it is placed in contact with one of the prepared pieces of gas meter skin in such a way that its most anterior tip lies just short of one end of the prepared skin and its lateral border just short of one of the long sides of the skin. (Fig. 29) So a prepared rubber surface meets a clean rubber surface, and the two will form a good bond. After the excess skin has been trimmed to within 2 or 3 mm. of the leading edge of the pad and of the medial border of the pad where it lies anterior to the band line (as in Fig. 32), the skin—the only visible

—side of the pad is cleaned with rubber solution and allowed to dry. When this is dry, the toe loop will be placed in position.

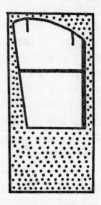

Fig. 29. Cell side down, the pad is placed in contact with the prepared side of the covering skin, taking care to leave spare covering material at the anterior, medial and lateral borders, with sufficient at the posterior border to allow for the remainder of the width of the band to be covered.

The toe loop was prepared during the stage of preparing the covering leathers. A length of prepared cover material was cut into a strip 16 mm. wide by at least 40 mm. more than the 'apparent' L. Loop measurement, the additional material having been left to provide anchoring tabs. The two marks on this strip which were furthest apart indicated the 'apparent' L. Loop measurement, and those nearest together towards the centre of the strip showed the position of the ends of the open cell insert; these four marks will show quite plainly through the coating of latex when it is dry.

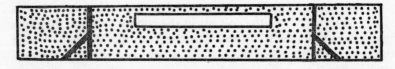

Fig. 30. The open cell insert in position on the loop material, the converging cuts are made to half-way across the marks indicating the 'apparent length' of the loop.

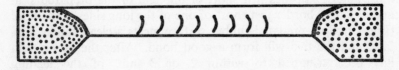

Fig. 31. The loop ready for attachment. The shaded area shows the prepared surface of the anchoring tabs.

Two *converging* cuts are made at an angle of approximately 45 deg. to end at the outside two marks and about half-way across the width of the material. The open cell insert, which will have been cut to size and cleaned with rubber solution, is now placed in the position marked by the two inside markings, with one edge at half the width of the strip of cover material (Fig. 30) and the centre portion of the strip is now folded over the insert and adhered edge to edge to enclose it completely, leaving at each end of the strip material which has not been folded to serve as anchoring tabs. (Fig. 31)

The loop is now placed with the adhesive anchorage areas in such a way that the folded edge of the loop faces outwards, and the ends of the folded edge occur *at* the points marked on the pad. Should the anchoring tabs prove to be long enough to tend to overlap each other, they should be turned back in such a way that the maximum possible area of each is in contact with the pad, surplus material being stuck together at right angles to the pad and trimmed off with scissors, resulting in a butted edge. (Fig. 32)

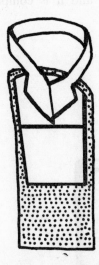

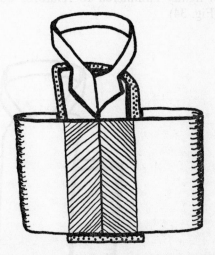

Fig. 32. The loop in position on the pad, the anterior and medial edges of the cover having been previously trimmed back.

Fig. 33. The band in position on the pad, with edges butted. Note that, at this stage, the untreated length of the band passes beneath the appliance, whilst the treated area is in contact with the clean rubber surfaces.

The uppermost surfaces of the anchoring tabs are now lightly coated with latex and the next operation is carried out taking care not to handle the wet latex.

A measured area of each end of the elastic webbing metatarsal band has been treated with latex. Working from the edge of the width of the pad and starting at the line on the pad which indicates the position of the leading edge of the band, one end of the rubberised part of the elastic webbing is secured to both the pad and the gas meter skin, holding the other end away from contact to avoid spoiling its adhesive surface. The untreated middle portion of the band is now passed *beneath* the half-completed appliance so that the other end of it may be butted with its partner to make, in effect, a continuous band around the forefoot. (Fig. 33)

At this stage excess covering material may be trimmed to within 2 or 3 mm. of the posterior edge of the band.

All of the adhesive areas are now cleaned with rubber solution (since they will have been subjected to much handling) and put aside to dry. When dry, the second piece of cover material is placed with its adhesive side towards the prepared surface of the appliance and pressed into place, working from the centre outwards. Now the excess material from the second cover is trimmed off, the appliance is lightly hammered to reinforce adhesion, and it is complete. (Fig. 34)

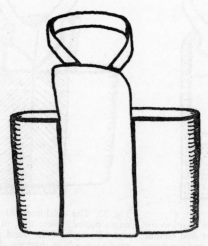

Fig. 34. The final cover having been trimmed, the appliance is now complete.

Single or Double Wing Extensions to the Metatarsal Pad

A wing to a metatarsal pad is an extension to one of its borders so that the full thickness of the pad continues sideways to behind the head of either the 1st or the 5th metatarsal; thus a single wing metatarsal pad will be 'Lateral Wing' or 'Medial Wing', although occasionally both wings are used on the same pad, so giving a 'Double Wing' pad. The idea behind this design of pad is to combine the action of the metatarsal pad with that of a protective crescent on the end of a shaft for a lesion on the 1st or 5th metatarsal head area. Since one of the functions of a protective crescent is to redistribute pressure from the lesion back on to the 'body' of the area of full thickness of the pad—in this case, from the metatarsal head area to the shaft—this will be found to work quite satisfactorily for the lateral wing (where the 5th metatarsal shaft lies over and more or less parallel to the insole of the shoe) but not for the medial wing. The angle at which the 1st metatarsal meets the insole of the shoe necessitates a very thick, impractical wing in order to fulfil its function by working on the area of flat insole of the shoe under the shaft of the 1st metatarsal. This is very small, leaving only the upper on which the shaft of the pad might work, distorting the shoe and reducing its effective depth to accommodate the rest of the foot. Where increased toe function of the 2nd, 3rd and 4th *can* be obtained, the metatarsal or lateral wing metatarsal pad will be effective without further modification in directing excess pressure away from *both* the 1st and 5th metatarso-phalangeal joints areas on to those of the 2nd, 3rd and 4th and their toes without the embarrassment of misshaping the shoe along its medial border. Where toe function in this area cannot be increased, a plantar cover for the 2nd, 3rd and 4th metatarso-phalangeal joint area or a lateral wing pad of this type will be found to be effective (see p. 82).

Should either a single or a double wing appliance be required, additional headings may be provided in the list on the measurement card—M.W. (medial wing) and Lat. W. (lateral wing).

In the case of a medial wing—should this be thought either desirable or effective—a measurement is taken on the foot transversely from the longitudinal reference line to the point at which the wing takes attachment at the medial edge of the main pad, recorded in brackets as a co-ordinate, and a further measurement is taken from the co-ordinate to the extreme medial edge of the wing. Applied to the metatarsal pad just dealt with, this might read M.W. (45)20. ((r)s in Fig. 35) It often happens that the anterior edge of the wing falls further forward than the leading edge of the band, and occasionally it may be required to be just behind the edge of the band. Applying the 'grid reference' principle, all measurements in the longitudinal plane which are anterior to the transverse reference line are recorded as positive, those posterior to it being negative—since the measurements must start from a common point and indication must be provided to show their direction. In the same manner, in the transverse plane, measurements originating from the longitudinal reference line are recorded as positive when they are medial to their starting point and negative when lateral. (Fig. 36)

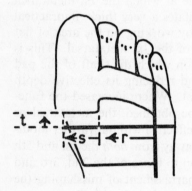

Fig. 35. The method of measuring the co-ordinate ('r' in the illustration) and from that the rest of the information for the medial wing. These readings would be recorded thus: M.W.(r)s plus t.

In the first case, where the edge of the wing was anterior to the transverse reference line, the distance from the edge of the band is measured and recorded thus: M.W. (r) s + t. (Fig. 35) For a lateral wing, a similar procedure is carried out, but there is no need for a co-ordinate as the wing takes attachment to the main body of the pad at the longitudinal reference line. (Fig. 37) It follows that this method may be extended to take in cover and other flat pads, even noting the location of cavities and other modifications just so long as two reference lines are in fixed positions at right angles to each other, 'bearings', as it were, being taken from them (e.g. see 'Plantar Cover Pads').

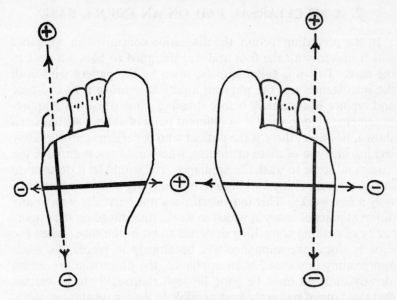

Fig. 36. The reference lines on a right and left foot showing how, in both cases, measurements in an anterior direction are positive, posterior negative, those going medial to the longitudinal reference line are positive, and those going lateral to it are negative.

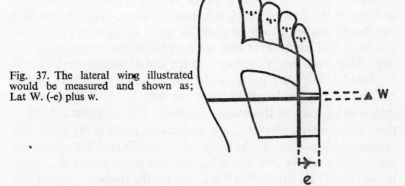

Fig. 37. The lateral wing illustrated would be measured and shown as; Lat W. (-e) plus w.

2. A METATARSAL PAD ON AN INSOLE BASE

In the preceding section, the discussion concerned an appliance which moved with the foot and was designed to be worn next to the skin. This was suitable to be worn by the patient with both the intelligence and the physical ability to remove it at bed-time and replace it accurately before dressing—one who would appreciate being able to wear it in different pairs of shoes. As has been shown, however, there is the patient who is perhaps unfortunately lacking in some of these attributes, who would not even have the 'common' sense to wash the appliance, and would let it degenerate into a most revolting looking and evil smelling affair in a matter of only a few weeks. This individual does not normally wear many different pairs of shoes in which to work, thus affording the opportunity of making something designed to go in the shoe; when the shoe is worn, the appliance will be already in place. As when appreciating any case for an appliance, the diagnostic procedure already outlined must be gone through thoroughly to be certain that this type of pad is the best possible in the circumstances. Also, the shoe must be considered as to whether or not it is suited to the intended action of the padding, and that it is the one worn to work every day and not just the 'Sunday best', worn for the visit to the surgery and for high days and holidays. The patient, the foot and the shoe having been taken into account, the 'insole' type of appliance may be thought to be the most advisable.

First, since the appliance is to fit in the shoe, it is necessary to gain an accurate outline of the insole—or flat part of the inside—of the shoe. If it is a new shoe this will not prove very difficult, but if, as is usually the case, it is an old one, it will have acquired an individual shape of its own which reflects quite accurately the activity of the foot to which it is host. A stock of clearly marked cardboard shapes which conform roughly to shoe sizes 1 to 12 will be found useful over and over again in this respect, and the one which most nearly conforms to the size of the shoe to be fitted is placed inside, any parts of the edges which fall short of the borders of the insole of the shoe are noted, whilst those which may overlap are—at this stage—ignored. The cardboard shape is then withdrawn and placed on a sheet of plain white foolscap; taking a ball-point pen, the shape of the cardboard is outlined on the paper, making due allowance for the edges which fell short in the shoe. (Fig. 38) Before the shape on the foolscap sheet is cut out, the name of the patient, the date and the case card number are written in at the heel to avoid confusion with any other templates, and the pattern is now placed in the shoe quite flat on the insole, a finger being pressed round its borders to show up any points at which it overlaps the edges of the insole. When the pattern is withdrawn the discrepancies will show up as ridges on the paper, and cutting along these lines where they exist will reduce it to the same size and shape as that of the insole of the shoe.

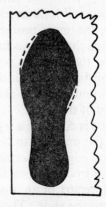

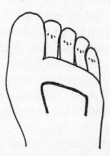

Fig. 38. The cardboard shape resting on the foolscap paper. The dotted line shows where extra material will be required, and it is the larger shape which is cut from the paper.

Fig. 39. The plantar surface of the foot marked up for a metatarsal pad on an insole base. Note that the markings are on the weight-bearing part of the skin only.

Since the appliance is to work using the shoe as its base, it *must* conform to the exact size and shape of its insole; if it were smaller or narrower, it would tend to move in the shoe during walking, if it were to overlap and take up more than the available space, it would exert pressure on the sides of the uppers, so reducing the total area available for toe function. Frequently there will be found to be a gap between the edge of the insole and the upper in an old or worn shoe; even when this is the case, the paper pattern is still made to the size of the insole, since otherwise the appliance and the foot in the shoe would widen the gap and cramp the toes.

The next stage in making the pattern is to mark the foot with the ball-point pen at the level of the 2nd, 3rd and 4th metatarsophalangeal joints, the marking being carried round into the 1st and 4th intermetatarsal spaces. (Fig. 39) A length of half-inch zinc oxide strapping is now attached to the upper surface of the paper pattern from the metatarsal area towards the heel and extending beyond by three or four inches. The pattern is then placed in position in the shoe and the strapping secured up the inside of the back of the heel so that it passes over the top and its end is free. This will serve the purpose of giving a light anchorage to the pattern when the foot is put into the shoe, and the free end will indicate if the pattern moves during walking. The shoe is now put on the bare foot and securely laced, the patient then being asked to stand up and walk for a minute or two. When the pattern is removed from the shoe, the mark of the foot will have transferred on to it as a slightly blurred double line, the most posterior of which showing the position of the mark when the shoe was first put on, the anterior giving a good guide as to the working position of the metatarso-phalangeal joints. It is this latter line which is to prove most useful in determining the positioning of the anterior, medial and lateral edges of the *full thickness* of the pad.

Next, a paper pattern of the pad to be used is cut from a separate piece of paper, allowing the thickness of the material to be used for skiving at the anterior, medial and lateral edges, with twice this for long skiving at the posterior edge. The purpose of long skiving at the posterior edge of any pad on the forepart of an insole is solely to aid the progression of the foot into the shoe. The paper pattern is marked with the name and relevant particulars of the patient, together with a note of the thickness and type of material to be used for the pad.

The choice of materials from which the base will be made rests with either regenerated leather, cork filled rubber sheeting, cork sheeting or a very stiff leather such as fleshing. Of these, the regenerated leather fibreboard is most commonly used, and with this material it will be found that one side of it is slightly 'fluffy' when compared with the other—it is this fluffy side to which the pad is attached.

The fibreboard is placed flat on the bench with its 'fluffy' side upwards, and on top of this goes the paper pattern (marked side up) of the insole of the shoe, the ball-point pen being used to outline its shape on the fibreboard. With the paper pattern still in position, the shape and markings for the pad are pricked through the paper pattern with the sharp point of the scissors to make a series of identifiable marks on the fibreboard, then the pattern is removed and the marks inked into a line which will indicate the exact position of the anterior, medial and lateral edges of the pad in relation to the rest of the insole shape. The insole shape, like the patterns, is marked at the heel with the name of the patient and relevant details, then cut from the sheet of fibreboard along the inside edge of the outline, the marked side coated with latex, and put aside to dry.

Next, the covering material is selected (usually a skiver leather), the flesh side—never the grain side—is marked with an outline of the paper pattern of the insole (marked side towards the flesh, and this time allowing about $\frac{1}{8}$ in. overlap all round), cut out, coated with latex and put aside to dry.

When placing a pad of closed cell sponge rubber on an insole base, the cell side should be towards the base, leaving the *skin side towards the foot*, this serving the purpose of giving a smooth finish to the surface of the appliance, thereby aiding the progression of the foot into the shoe as well as giving the pad a particularly firm attachment to the base by virtue of the increased area of adhesion offered by the cell side of the rubber. With this in mind, the paper pattern of the pad is placed with its marked side uppermost on the skin side of a sheet of closed cell sponge rubber of the appropriate thickness, and the outline of the shape of the pattern is marked on the skin. Again, the name and relevant details are written inside the outline, which is then cut out ready for skiving.

Since the aim is to present as smooth a surface of the appliance as possible to the foot, the skiving is carried out on the cell side. If ordinary skiving is used, the result will be a very wrinkled skived edge being presented for adhesion to the base and stress being caused in the skin surface. In the illustration (Fig. 40) it will be seen that ABC is an isosceles triangle, CA being equal to CB. Fig. 41 shows that AB is wrinkled and it is stretching CB (since

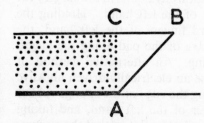

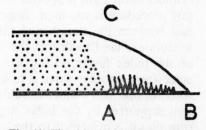

Fig. 40. The full thickness of the pad (cell side) adhered to the base, with a straight 45 degree skive.

Fig. 41. The skived edge of the pad in Fig. 40 stuck to the base, showing wrinkles of densely packed material in the area of adhesion AB and tensile stress at CB.

the material is rubber) which is curved convexly; from this, it is obvious that the curved line CB has become longer than the distance of A to B along the insole base also, the material at CB will tend to return to its original length, pulling AB off the insole base. The object is therefore to lengthen AB to equal CB. If the skiving is concave instead of straight, this will achieve the desired result, at the same time as disposing of some surplus material.

Sponge rubber, when bent, distorts more markedly than many other materials, so if it is cut or skived when it is bent, the resultant cut or skive will reflect this distortion quite accurately. Should a border of the pad be bent lengthwise over a cylinder and a straight lengthwise skive be carried out whilst it is held in this position (Fig. 42) when the rubber is allowed to lie flat again the skive will be found to be concave (Fig. 43). The most convenient

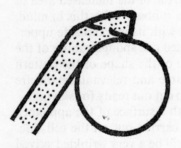
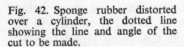
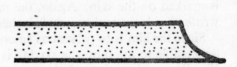

Fig. 42. Sponge rubber distorted over a cylinder, the dotted line showing the line and angle of the cut to be made.

Fig. 43. The edge of the cut rubber, when allowed to lie flat, will reflect the circumference of the cylinder on which it was skived.

cylinder of the right proportions readily available in the surgery for this procedure is the index finger of the left hand. Holding the pad between the thumb and third fingers of the left hand, the scissors are used to distort the edge of the pad along the length of the index finger during skiving. An alternative method of achieving a concave skive is to use an electrically-driven abrasive wheel of one inch diameter, holding the edge of the sponge rubber well supported by the index finger of the left hand, and taking care that it is presented to the wheel quite flat so that the circumference of the wheel will be reflected in the skive (the work must be well supported, undistorted, and the cutting facets of the wheel allowed to do the major part of the effort). (Figs. 44 and 45)

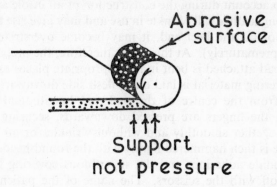

Fig. 44. The edge of the sponge rubber, well supported, being skived by the abrasive wheel (which turns anti-clockwise).

The cell side of the pad is to have normal skiving at the anterior, medial and lateral edges; that is to say that the edges of full thickness of the pad are to be the same distance from the edge of the pad itself as the thickness of material used, and these edges are given concave skiving. The posterior edge, however, has long skiving and therefore does not present the problem which required the normal skiving to be concave. The cell side of the pad is cleaned with rubber solution after skiving, and when dry is placed so that its edges of full thickness coincide with the markings on the prepared surface of the insole base. Working with the fingers pressing down from the centre of the skin side towards the edges, the pad is moulded on to the base. The skin side of the pad is then cleaned with rubber solution, taking the solution over the edges and on to the dry latex surface of the base, the whole then being allowed to dry.

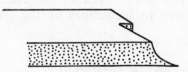

Fig. 45. After skiving on the wheel, the shape of its circumference is found to have been cut into the edge of the sponge rubber.

It will be observed that the insole of a shoe, although fairly flat transversely, is curved longitudinally at several points, notably just anterior to the heel seating, again at the point just anterior to the waist, and again towards the toe-box. Unless these curves are taken into account during the construction of an insole appliance, the covering leather will wrinkle in use and may give rise to lesions on the foot (at the heel end, it may become overstretched and wear out prematurely). At this stage, therefore, the prepared base with the pad attached is bent in the appropriate places as the prepared covering material is laid on it, flesh side downwards. Again working from the centre of the pad and longitudinal mid-line outwards, the fingers are pressed downwards, securing the two surfaces together smoothly and without wrinkles or air bubbles. The insole is then hammered lightly with the round-headed mallet to consolidate adhesion, and the superfluous covering leather is trimmed off with the scissors. The name of the patient is now covered up inside the appliance, so it is marked on the under side if this is not to be covered as well.

Since the materials have been handled extensively during the process of construction, the grain side of the leather cover should now be polished after cleaning with a little soft soap, both to add finish to the appearance and to aid progression of the foot into the shoe.

3. A 'DUDLEY MORTON' PROP

Dudley Morton's Syndrome

A syndrome is a collection of signs and symptoms; Dudley Morton's Syndrome may be thought of as consisting of three:

1. Thickening of the head of the 2nd metatarsal.
2. Thickening of the shaft of the 2nd metatarsal.
3. Pain at the base of the 2nd metatarsal.

The syndrome may occur for one or other of many different reason or reasons, but Dudley Morton* first grouped them together and noticed that they were all due to inefficiency of the 1st metatarsal which may be:

A short 1st metatarsal.
Metatarsus Primus Elevatus (elevated 1st metatarsal).
Metatarsus Primus Varus.
Hypermobile 1st metatarsal.
Posteriorly placed sesamoids.

* *The Human Foot: Its Evolution, Physiology and Functional Disorders*, by Dudley J. Morton. Cambridge University Press, 1935.

Dudley Morton found that, for some of these conditions which could lead to the Syndrome (the signs of which usually include pressure lesions on the areas of the plantar surface of the 1st interphalangeal joint and at that of the 2nd metatarso-phalangeal joint), the way to alleviate it was to make the 1st metatarsal do its fair share of weight-bearing. Since it was designed to take one-third of the weight shared by the five metatarsals, any inefficiency of the 1st is bound to cause overloading of one or more of the others (when D.M. Syndrome is present, there is no pressure lesion on the 1st metatarso-phalangeal joint area). With this in view, he designed an insole which incorporated a pad, the full thickness (or operative part) of which extended from the inter-phalangeal joint of the first toe to a point half or two-thirds the length of the shaft of the 1st metatarsal towards its base, the width conforming to that of the 1st metatarsal. This type of insole was not intended to restrict movement in the 1st metatarso-phalangeal joint, but to increase the efficiency of the 1st metatarsal in one of two ways:

1. By 'filling in the gap', as it were, between the 1st metatarsal and the ground. 'Bringing the ground up' to the 1st metatarsal segment.
2. By having the effect of re-directing weight forward, thus apparently extending the length of the metatarsal.

One or other—or a combination of both—of these will directly benefit five conditions by the methods of action already described:

1. The short 1st metatarsal.
2. Metatarsus Primus Elevatus.
3. Metatarsus Primus Varus.
4. Posteriorly placed sesamoids.
5. Hallux Rigidus (if used in conjunction with other measures which are designed to restrict movement at the M.P. joint).

Since the efficiency of the first metatarsal is increased, the pain of the Syndrome will decrease, resulting in improved function of the foot.

A 'Dudley Morton' Prop on an Insole

This is an adhesive felt pad which owes its origin to the Dudley Morton Insole; the thickness and density of the adhesive pad will depend upon the degree of defect present. Normal skiving is used at the anterior, medial and lateral borders, with long skiving at the posterior end, and both the pad and its strapping is used in such a way as to permit a full range of movement at the metatarso-phalangeal joint. This is achieved by attaching the anterior end of the pad to the plantar surface of the first toe, and dorsiflexing the toe fully whilst attaching the pad to the areas of the metatarso-phalangeal joint and the metatarsal shaft; whilst still in this position, the lateral strap is attached (as the skin is under tension). The medial strap, however, should be attached when the toe is in the rest—or even the slightly plantar flexed—position, since the skin in this part of the foot is under tension when the toe is in this position, and the strapping will not therefore have any restricting effect when in use. The anterior transverse anchoring strap is then passed round the toe, and lastly the posterior strap is placed in position again when the toe is dorsiflexed. The result of this method of application of pad and strapping is that the toe is un-impeded in movement whilst the metatarsal is assisted by the pad. (Fig. 46) The fact that, whatever position the toe is in, one or other of the longitudinal straps will be wrinkled, although giving a less tidy appearance, is of no greater consequence than just giving an indication that the strapping has been applied with due regard to its proper function: the wrinkles will only follow the normal skin creases. A test as to whether or not the pad and strapping have been correctly applied is to dorsiflex the toe. If the dressing

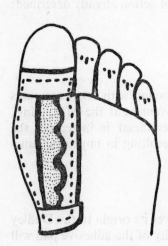

Fig. 46. The adhesive felt 'Dudley Morton' prop strapped in position on the foot at rest. The lateral strap will be slightly wrinkled, whilst the medial strap will not when the toe is in this position.

has been incorrectly applied, the posterior end will break free from the skin or else give undue tension to the skin at this area. Should the patient be allowed to leave the surgery with the dressing in this condition, on the next visit it will be found that:

1. The pad has not fulfilled its function, there being no improvement of pressure signs or symptoms.
2. If it stayed in position, there will be found to be a series of stress marks on the skin under the posterior end of the dressing. These are often mistaken as showing plaster idiosyncrasy, but closer examination will reveal that they occur only under one part of the dressing and not beneath the whole area covered by the plaster mass.

Having successfully used the 'Dudley Morton' Prop in adhesive materials, an appliance may be considered. There is the choice of making a removable appliance or an insole. The removable type will be discussed under the heading 'Chairside Appliances'. The first step in making a 'Dudley Morton' Prop on an insole base is to take a paper pattern of the insole of the shoe in the manner previously described, then the foot is marked with the ball-point pen at the interphalangeal joint of the first toe and along the line of the 1st intermetatarsal space. These lines indicate the position of the borders (anterior and lateral) of the pad, and due account must be taken of the thickness of material to be used in arriving at them. The medial border will be that of the medial edge of the insole itself, and the posterior edge, if marked on the foot, will not transfer to the paper pattern since it is not a part of the skin which is normally weight-bearing. The patient is then asked to stand up and walk for a few minutes, and the resultant marks on the paper pattern will form the starting point from which to make a pattern of the pad at a later stage, remembering that its medial border conforms to that of the medial border of the insole pattern at this point.

The base material is selected and cut out according to the pattern as described earlier, marked with the positions of the edges of the pad (as well as with the name of the patient), the top surface coated with latex—if regenerated leather sheeting is being used—and put aside to dry. The cover material is selected, but when cutting out according to the paper pattern, although allowing the $\frac{1}{8}$ in. all round, extra material over and above this must be left at the medial edge of the pad. (Fig. 47) The flesh side of the cover material, having been marked with the name of the patient, is then brushed with latex and laid aside to dry. Using the paper pattern of the full thickness of the pad, marked side up, the closed cell sponge rubber of thickness appropriate to the degree of defect is marked with the outline on the skin side, making allowance for the skiving, cut out, given a short concave skiving on its anterior and lateral edges, a long straight skiving at its posterior edge and no skiving on the medial border, marked with the name of the patient, and then cleaned on its cell side with rubber solution.

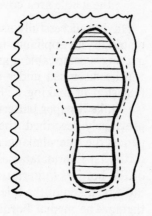

Fig. 47. The paper pattern, resting marked side towards the flesh side of the covering leather, outlined as described with ⅛ in. all round except at the medial border of the pad, where the full thickness of the pad (as well as the ⅛ in.) is allowed.

When all three parts of the appliance—the base, the cover and the pad—are dry, the pad is adhered to the base cell side down with its full thickness in the position marked, and the skin side and edges (including the unskived medial edge) are cleaned with rubber solution. When this is dry, the covering material is stuck to the base and pad, taking care to maintain the toe and heel spring, and to see that the extra material allowed at the medial edge of the pad falls into the right position. (Fig. 48)

The purpose of allowing extra material at the medial edge of the pad is to have sufficient to be able to cover it, but if this material is just 'flopped' into position, folds will be found at either end of the edge of the pad (if not elsewhere as well) which will add extra thickness to the width of the appliance as well as spoiling its appearance. The procedure, then, is to attach the covering mate-

Fig. 48. A medial view, with the insole tilted up at the lateral border, showing the flap of the extra covering leather at the medial border of the pad. At this stage, all the extra 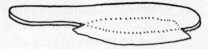 covering material has been trimmed off with the exception of the flap, which is in the same plane as the insole. The outline of the pad can just be discerned.

rial to this edge of the pad by pleating it with the back of a blade of a pair of scissors; this is done by first attaching the material at the centre of the length of the pad, then at either end, resulting in two half lengths of the material remaining unattached. These are each divided in half by pressing the back of the blade of the scissors on the cover material to make it contact the edge of the pad, the remaining sections are each divided in half in the same way, and so on until all the cover material is attached. The result will now be that the edge at this point has a slightly corrugated appearance, so the top surface of the pad is gently tapped with the round-headed mallet, then the edge itself, this having the effect of securing the whole of the edge of the pad to the whole of the flesh side of the covering material, resulting in a smooth finish on the grain side of the leather. Finally, the superfluous cover material is trimmed off, and the name of the patient recorded on the under side of the insole unless it is intended to cover this side with perhaps a split suède for extra finish.

4. SOME REMOVABLE PLANTAR COVER PADS

A plantar cover pad is one which has its full thickness extending from over the bases of the proximal phalanges of the 1st, 2nd, 3rd, 4th and 5th toes to a point on the metatarsals which is dependent upon the material used for the pad, and from the medial side of the medial sesamoid to the lateral side of the weight-bearing area of the 5th metatarso-phalangeal joint. Normal skiving is used on the anterior, medial and lateral edges, with long skiving on the posterior edge. (Fig. 49) The purpose of the pad is to make up for deficiency in the superficial fascia at the weight-bearing area of the metatarsals by:

1. Artificial cushioning. This depending upon the material to be used.

2. Thermal insulation, or protection against the heat generated by friction where the natural protection is inadequate. This could be produced very adequately with polyurethane foam.

Modifications may be made in certain materials to afford protection for a lesion or lesions or to increase the load taken by certain of the M.P. joints.

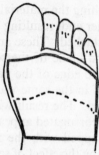

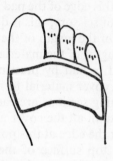

Fig. 49. The basic shape of a plantar cover pad before modification for its specific purpose. The dotted line indicates the posterior end of the weight-bearing part of the forefoot.

Fig. 50. The open cell cover pad in position.

The 'Cushion' Plantar Cover Pad

When the plantar cover pad is being used to provide the first of the two types of protection mentioned, it is made of open cell material. As was seen in the discussion on open cell sponge rubber (see p. 23), if this material is completely sealed in it will act as an air pillow—as one large bubble of air—and this effect could be achieved to a limited extent by covering the pad in completely with strapping. Should this be done with a pad of a shape as shown in the illustration (Fig. 49), the air already contained under the weight-bearing areas of the metatarso-phalangeal joints will be forced into the posterior, non-weight-bearing, part of the pad, so the only benefit which the dressing will impart to the foot will be that afforded by the very thin layer of material remaining between the foot and the footwear; a degree of thermal insulation. With this in mind, then, the cover pad which is to be of open cell sponge rubber to act as a cushion is shaped to conform only to the shape of the weight-bearing area. (Fig. 50)

Having found that this type of padding achieves the best

obtainable results in adhesive materials in any particular case, and there being no immediate prospect of marked improvement in the condition of the foot by continuing with these methods, an appliance will be considered. Fig. 50 shows the shape of the open cell sponge rubber which would be used either on an insole base or as a removable pad, but on the removable pad the shape presents some difficulty of attachment to the metatarsal band. The posterior edge of the pad at the 2nd, 3rd and 4th metatarsal shafts (depending on the metatarsal formula) would often fall anterior to the leading edge of the band, gaining no attachment to it at all. A digital loop as the sole means of attachment of the appliance to the foot might tend to cut in on the interdigital webbing, causing discomfort and perhaps breaks in the skin surface. The solution to this problem, then, is to provide an anchorage to the metatarsal band by splicing the open cell cushion pad with closed cell sponge rubber, the shape of which will bring the combined outline to that shown in Fig. 49. As the closed cell material will be posterior to the metatarsal heads, it cannot affect either the function of the foot or that of the pad as long as its thickness does not exceed that of the open cell cushion.

The measurement principle may be applied to the removable plantar cover using the same basis as that for the metatarsal pad, the vertical list of measurements on the left of the card referring to the open cell pad and those alongside, and on the right referring to the closed cell anchoring material. As with the metatarsal and single wing pads, with the exception of the length and width of the pad, all measurements originate from the reference lines, which are placed as before. The measurements required then are:

The *width* of the pad (and of its posterior border in the case of the closed cell part).
The *length* of the basic rectangle.
Two or more readings for the *band* to *tip* at the *mid-line* side of the longitudinal reference.
The *band* to *tip* at the *lateral border* (one on the longitudinal reference line, another at the lateral border).

Where any of the last two readings are posterior to the band, they are recorded as minus, and any transverse readings lateral to the longitudinal reference line will also be minus. Measurements under the heading 'B.T. (mid.)' will require co-ordinates, in much the same way as with the medial wing metatarsal pad, so also will co-ordinates be required for the B.T.(lat.) readings (see Figs. 35, 36 and 37). All the other measurements are taken in the same way as those of the metatarsal pad, and from the information so collected and recorded (Figs. 51 and 53) the pad may be constructed in the two materials.

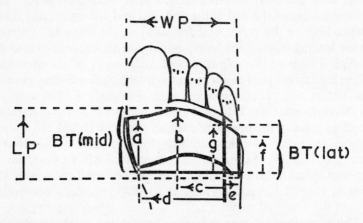

Fig. 51. Showing how the co-ordinates—in brackets—and the positive and negative signs are used to give the direction of measurement. The open cell part of the pad is measured from the reference lines as illustrated, and would be recorded thus:
B.T. (mid.) (c)b, (d)a.
B.T. (lat.) g, (-e)f.

Translation of the measurements. Thinking first of the *open cell pad*, a rectangle which represents the measurements L.P. by W.P. is marked out on open cell sponge rubber, and the highest B.T.(mid.) measurement (here b) is used to give the transverse reference line. Then the B.T.(lat.) co-ordinate (here e) is used to give the distance of the longitudinal reference line from the lateral edge of the rectangle. Now the anterior edge of the pad must be marked in, using the first measurement under B.T.(lat.) (g) to indicate its position on the longitudinal reference line, that at the co-ordinate for the placing of the meeting point of the anterior and lateral edges of the pad (f); under B.T.(mid.), the first measurement (c) gives the co-ordinate and measurement of the anterior edge of the pad (b) in the region of the second metatarsal, and the second for the placing at the medial edge of the pad at the transverse reference line (d) a. More co-ordinates and measurements may be recorded if necessary, if the curve of the edge of the pad is sufficiently complex, although the metatarsal formula and the readings related to the longest and shortest metatarsals constitute important additional information in relation to the curvature of the edge. Since the cover pad lies over all the five metatarsal heads, the relative size of each will be of assistance in plotting the shape of the anterior edge of the pad—the first metatarsal head will occupy one-third of the width of the pad, whilst the other four will take up one-quarter each of the remainder. Bearing in mind that the measurement for the fifth metatarsal—representative in width of the four lesser metatarsals—is already recorded under the co-ordinate at B.T.(lat.), mark off accordingly on the anterior edge of the rectangle. (Fig. 52)

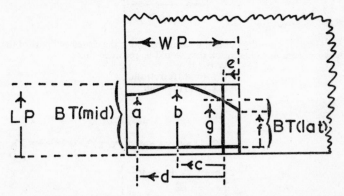

Fig. 52. Translation of the measurements on to open cell material. Having drawn the basic rectangle, the reference lines are marked, and from these the anterior and lateral borders of the pad are calculated and marked. The material is then cut from the sheet along the markings of the lateral and anterior edges of the *pad*, the medial and posterior edges of the *rectangle*.

Now the basic rectangle from the measurements taken as in Fig. 53 is marked on the skin side of the *closed cell* sponge rubber sheet in the manner shown in Fig. 54, the shape of the pad is marked in and cut from the sheet of material with the anterior edge skived—with normal skiving—on its *cell* side.

Splicing the two materials. The skived anterior edge of the closed cell pad is cleaned with rubber solution; *only* the skived edge is so treated, should any of the solution stray on to the full thickness of the material, it should be powdered with a little talcum when dry to spoil its adhesive properties. An area surrounding the transverse reference line on the open cell pad is cleaned with rubber

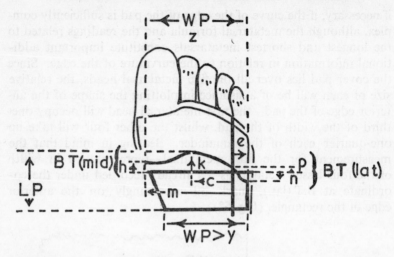

Fig. 53. Here the co-ordinates and measurements for the closed cell part of the pad are shown. From this illustration they would be recorded thus:

W.P. z > y
B.T. (mid.) (c)k, (m)h.
B.T. (lat.) p, (-e)-n.

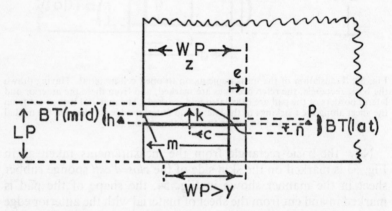

Fig. 54. Translation of the measurements on to the skin side of the closed cell sponge rubber.

solution and, when both are dry, the prepared anterior edge of the closed cell pad is placed in contact with the prepared surface of the open cell pad so that:

1. The lateral edges of the two materials form a straight line.
2. The longitudinal reference line on the closed cell pad appears to be both continuous and straight with as much as can be seen of it on the surface of the open cell material.
3. As in 2, so with the transverse reference line.

Only the skived edge of the closed cell pad is allowed to adhere to the open cell surface (since only this part of the closed cell material has an effectively clean rubber surface, the remainder will not gain a firm bond), and the two materials, now united in 'mousetrap' fashion (Fig. 55), are placed marked side down on a flat surface, and the surplus open cell material skived off with scissors cutting in the plane of the flat surface so that the whole area of full thickness of the closed cell material is exposed, leaving only the skived edge attached to the open cell pad. (Fig. 56) The result is now one large pad consisting of the two materials spliced together. Turning this so that the skin side of the closed cell section is uppermost, the transverse reference line should be found to run straight across the two materials in an unbroken straight line which should be parallel to the posterior edge of the pad.

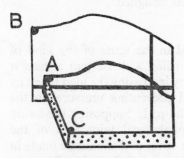

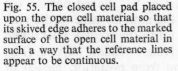

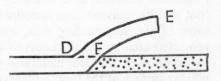

Fig. 55. The closed cell pad placed upon the open cell material so that its skived edge adheres to the marked surface of the open cell material in such a way that the reference lines appear to be continuous.

Fig. 56. A sectional view of the two pads with the skin side of the closed cell pad (shaded) down on a flat surface. The surplus open cell material is skived off with the scissors held flat, cutting through DF (dotted line).

The medial edge of the pad is now shaped by cutting from the top of the medial edge of the closed cell section to that of the open cell (Fig. 55, A to B, forming the medial edge of the combined pad BC). The pad of combined materials is now ready for underskiving, using normal skiving all round except at the posterior edge, which has long skiving. The under, or unmarked side, is now cleaned with rubber solution and laid aside to dry.

As with all these types of removable appliances, the materials which will have latex treatment will have been prepared before attention is paid to the pad, and when both these and the pad are dry, the pad is placed cell side down on to the prepared surface of one of the pieces of covering leather, adhered firmly, and the surplus free edge at the anterior and medial edges as far as the leading edge of the band may be trimmed to about $\frac{1}{4}$ in. of the edge of the pad. The elastic webbing band is now placed in position with the two edges butted in the same manner as with the removable metatarsal pad appliance (Fig. 33), and when these are stuck to the pad and the underlying covering material, and have dried after cleaning with rubber solution, the final cover is put into place. The appliance is then hammered lightly, *omitting* the area of open cell material, and the edges trimmed off to within just over $\frac{1}{8}$ in. of the pad and band. Care should be scrupulously taken with this type of pad not to trim too close to the edges of the open cell pad in case the effect of providing an airtight compartment for the open cell material is lost, together with all the cushioning effect for which the appliance was designed.

The Protective Plantar Cover Pad

The term 'protective' is here used in the sense of the kind of protection afforded to a lesion by using a dense pad *around* it (not over it), redistributing pressure by increasing the load taken by some of the surrounding area, and preventing pressure on the protected area by the thickness of the pad. Supposing the lesion to occur over the 3rd metatarso-phalangeal joint area of the plantar surface of the foot, a plantar cover pad should be made in $\frac{3}{16}$ in. or $\frac{5}{16}$ in. felt with a crescentic or 'U' shaped portion cut out so that the open end occurs at the anterior edge of the pad, and the full thickness of the pad is up to the medial, lateral and posterior edges of the lesion, with skiving extending beyond. (Fig. 57) This pad will protect the lesion from posterior, medial or lateral excess pressure by its thickness (which stands above it), and by its area taking the redistributed pressure and spreading it over the 1st, 2nd, 4th and 5th metatarso-phalangeal joints.

This pad may be translated into either a removable appliance or into an insole. Of these alternatives the removable pad is preferable (other factors previously mentioned having been taken

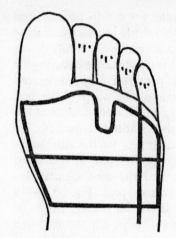

Fig. 57. A 'U-ed' plantar cover pad marked on the foot.

into account); since it moves with the foot it should stay in closer proximity to the lesion and so give it better protection. A first step in making the removable protective cover pad as an appliance is to apply the measurement principle to it. (Fig. 58)

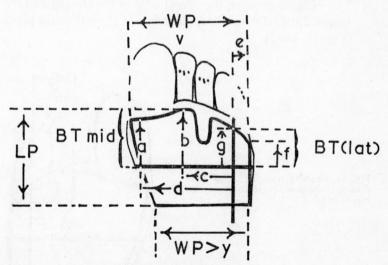

Fig. 58. The measurement principle, applied to this pad, would yield readings (apart from LP and WP, which are taken in the usual way) thus:
B.T. (mid.) (c)b, (d)a.
B.T. (lat.) g, (-e)f.

The name of the patient and other relevant details having been recorded at the top of the card, the object behind the measurements is to arrive at the basic rectangle within which lie the limits of the pad. Thus the length of the pad (L.P.) is the distance between the most anterior tip of the pad and the posterior edge, measured parallel to the fourth intermetatarsal space. The width of the pad is the distance between the most medial and the lateral edges of the pad when measured parallel to the leading edge of the metatarsal band (which runs at right angles to the 4th intermetatarsal space). The posterior edge of the pad is measured from the lateral to the medial edges, and the measurement recorded in the same way as with the metatarsal pad. Fig. 58 shows that the B.T.(mid.) measurements are taken, as before, from the two co-ordinates, one under the 'highest' edge on the mid-line side of the longitudinal reference, the other at the medial edge of the pad at the transverse reference line (d), the B.T.(lat.) measurements being taken as before. So the position of the band relative to the anterior edge of the pad has been noted, together with information about the shape and size of the pad with the exception of the cut-out portion of the lesion; for these, three measurements are required:

1. The distance between the lateral edge of the cut-out and the longitudinal reference line, measured in the transverse plane (Fig. 59, Lat r).

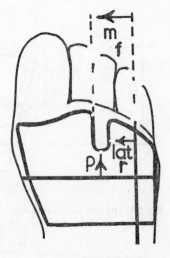

Fig. 59. Showing how the 'U-ed' portion is measured in relation to the reference lines.

2. The distance between the medial edge of the cut-out and the longitudinal reference line, in the transverse plane (M f).
3. The distance between the proximal edge of the cut-out and the transverse reference in the longitudinal plane (PB p).

Measurements for the metatarsal band are taken in the same way as for a metatarsal pad on a band. A toe loop may be used if required (in which case the measurements will be taken accordingly), but this is not usually necessary since the pad rarely has any tendency to move posteriorly during walking, as the weight of the patient tends to anchor it in position throughout the stage where the forefoot is in contact with the ground, unlike the metatarsal pad, which tends to be squeezed posteriorly. Where the occasional patient does experience difficulty may be during the process of donning hosiery, and it is mainly for these cases that a toe loop may be found to be useful.

Using the measurements and information recorded on the card, the appliance is made on the same principle as before. On the skin side of the closed cell sponge rubber of appropriate thickness the basic rectangle is marked out, together with the line for the leading edge of the metatarsal band (the transverse reference). The B.T.(lat.) co-ordinate is used to find the longitudinal reference line, and the

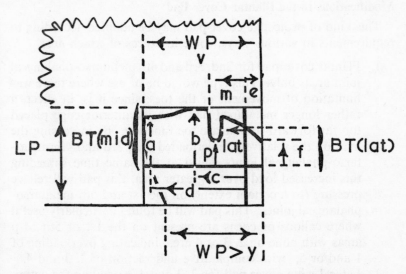

Fig. 60. The skin side of the closed cell material marked with the rectangle, reference lines and shape of the pad with the 'U-ed' cavity.

metatarsal formula and the B.T.(lat.) readings are used together to arrive at and mark the shape of the anterior edge of the pad without the U-ed cavity. This is the stage at which the shape, size and position of the cavity is found and marked; the measurement PB p indicates that its posterior (or proximal) edge lies p mm. from the transverse reference, so a line is drawn parallel to and p mm. forward of the band line. Similarly, the measurement M f results in a line being drawn parallel to and f mm. from the medial side of the longitudinal reference line, and again, Lat r gives a line parellel to and r mm. from the same starting point. The result of these markings is shown in the illustration (Fig. 60), and gives the position, shape and size of the cavity. The measurement for the width of the pad (WP v> y) showed that the posterior border measured y mm. from the lateral edge of the pad—or rectangle—so a line is ruled from that point to the point at which the anterior edge of the pad meets the medial edge, this line now representing the medial border of the pad.

The closed cell sponge rubber material for the pad is now fully marked up and ready to be cut out, underskiving all the edges. The procedure from this point is essentially the same as that for a metatarsal pad on a band.

Modifications to the Plantar Cover Pad

This kind of protective cover pad may be adapted according to requirements in various ways, some instances of which are:

1. Plantar cover pad for 2nd, 3rd and 4th metatarso-phalangeal joint areas only. This type would be of use where there was limitation of movement of the toes, since it is, in effect, a rather longer metatarsal pad with its anterior edge placed too far forward to increase toe function. By increasing the load on the relatively underloaded 2nd, 3rd and 4th metar-tarso-phalangeal joints whilst at the same time spreading this increased load over a greater area, this pad will relieve pressure (to a certain extent) on the 1st and 5th metatarso-phalangeal joints. This pad will be found particularly useful where callous or corns are present on the 1st or 5th M-p areas with none on 2, 3 or 4 area, indicating overloading of 1 and/or 5, with comparative underaction of 2, 3 and 4.

2. Lateral wing cover pad for 2, 3 and 4, extending the action of the above pad to accentuate the protection of the 5th

metatarso-phalangeal joint by taking some of the pressure on the 5th metatarsal shaft.

3. Plantar cover pad with a 'Dudley Morton' type extension at the shaft of the 1st proximal phalanx.

The measurement principle may be easily adapted to these and any other modifications of plantar padding.

5. PLANTAR COVER PADS ON INSOLE BASES

The 'Cushion' Plantar Cover Pad

The purpose of this pad is to cushion the area of the ball of the foot, and if a removable cover cushion appliance is thought inadvisable for a patient, the need may arise to translate the pad into an appliance on an insole base.

First, then, a paper pattern is taken of the insole of the shoe in the same manner as that used for metatarsal or similar pads on insoles. Next, the edges of the position of the open cell material cushion pad (as it would be in position) are marked on the foot with the ball-point pen. Now since these edges will be on the fringes of the weight-bearing area of the ball of the foot, care must be exercised over the marking; if the line is *beyond* the weight-bearing area at any point it will not transfer to the paper pattern when the patient walks on it, whereas if the line is too far *within* the area, the pad will be too small to achieve its fullest effect. So the mark on the foot is made as a *broad* one on the edges of the area, and some of the width of it will not transfer to the pattern.

When the shape of the outline of the pad in position while the patient was walking has been obtained on the insole pattern, it is made into a paper template of the pad, which is then translated into the pad itself in open cell sponge rubber of the appropriate thickness, and rounded at the edges (rather than skived, which is usually unnecessary with this material). The material to be used for the base is marked in accordance with the insole pattern, cut out, and the position of the pad marked in as previously described. Here it is vital to see that *no* edge of the pad coincides with the edge of the insole base, since the open cell sponge rubber is to be hermetically sealed (unless the shoe is an outstandingly bad fit in width, the edges of the weight-bearing area of the ball of the foot should not coincide with the edge of the insole in any case). (Fig. 61) The leather to be used for covering the appliance—skiver, perhaps, persian lamb or glacé kid—is marked on the flesh side

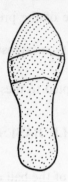

Fig. 61. The markings on the paper insole template for the 'cushion' cover pad may run off the medial and lateral edges where they have been transferred from the foot. Where this is the case, medial and lateral edges are marked in (shown as dotted lines) about ¼ in. from the edges of the insole before the paper pattern for the pad is made.

and cut out, allowing about ½ in. all round the edges of the paper template, then both the top surface of the insole base and the flesh side of the covering material are coated with latex and laid aside to dry, while the under side of the pad is cleaned with rubber solution.

When the prepared surfaces are dry, the pad is placed in the position marked on the base, and its top surface cleaned with rubber solution. When this is dry, the covering skin is placed over the base and pad (with its rubberised flesh side downwards) and attached along the longitudinal centre, establishing the heel and toe springs, then outwards towards the medial and lateral borders. Care should be taken not to squash the pad during this operation, as the object is to *trap the air within the pad*, not to squeeze it out. The whole is now hammered—with the exception of the pad area—and the surplus covering material trimmed off. The grain surface of the covering leather is now cleaned and polished, and the appliance is complete. To test the cushioning action, if one end of the pad is palpated (gently, when the adhesives are still fresh), the other should distend, thus showing that the action of a single cell of air is complete and without leaks.

The Protective Cover Pad

The purpose of this pad was described in the discussion on removable pads. Since the marks for the anterior edge of the pad and a little of the medial and lateral edges are all that will transfer to the paper pattern, these are all that are marked on the foot; any 'U-ed' cavity may also be marked. The shape of the posterior end of the pad will allow for its full thickness to extend to about two-thirds the length of the shafts of the metatarsals, so this is allowed for when the paper template of the pad is made. The pad itself is made of closed cell sponge rubber, and if it is intended to be a full cover pad—that is, if it is to cover the areas of the 1st and 5th metatarso-phalangeal joints as well as those of the rest—then the medial and lateral edges should not be skived at all, for the same reason as that which applied to the medial edge of the 'Dudley Morton' prop on an insole base. Apart from these considerations, the procedure in making any of the protective cover pads on an insole base is the same as that already described.

6. A VALGUS REST PAD

In approaching the treatment of a valgus foot, it must first be decided what a valgus foot is, and what is causing the trouble. As far as the skeletal structures are concerned, the calcaneum is rotated medially about its longitudinal axis so that its lateral tuberosity is raised and the talus, being locked between the tibia and fibula and so unable to follow this rotation, tilts forwards and downwards so that its head pushes the navicular forwards and downwards, this having the same effect on all three cuneiforms. The result of the movement of the cuneiforms is to push the first three metatarsals forwards and, as they cannot move downwards because of their contact with the ground, to effect a rotation of the 1st metatarsal about its longitudinal axis so that its lateral border is raised; the phalanges of the 1st, 2nd and 3rd toes are pushed forwards, those of the 1st following the direction of the rotation of their metatarsal. Thus, the medial longitudinal arch is lowered and the medial side of the foot considerably lengthened. On the lateral side of the foot, the cuboid is said to take a slight forwards and downwards movement (although most of the thrust of this has been taken and transmitted by the navicular) passing on what there is of this movement to the 4th and 5th metatarsals and their toes; but it should be emphasised that this tendency on the lateral border of the foot can only be slight in comparison with that of the medial border, since (with the exception of the cuboid) the bones of the lateral side of the foot are normally in contact with the ground on weight-bearing and the forwards and downwards movement, transmitted mainly by the talus, is most effective on the medial border of the foot.

Thus, in a valgus foot, there is a pronounced lengthening of the foot on its medial border without a comparable change at the lateral, with the result that the whole foot is swung into the valgus position and the forefoot, when considered in relation to the rotated calcaneum, is supinated. The effect of all this on the ligamentous structures is most marked at the inferior calcaneo-navicular (or 'spring') ligament, which is placed under considerable stress producing pain in the area, and the plantar fascia as well as some of the interosseous ligaments are also stretched and painful. The foot will be inverted by the synergistic action of the tibialis anterior and posterior, assisted in some respects by the flexors hallucis and digitorum longus and digitorum brevis, whilst the evertors are slackened.

The foregoing is an outline of what happens *within* a valgus foot. The outward or *visible* signs are:

1. The lateral deviation of the forefoot, with the lengthening of the foot on its medial border.
2. The unusual prominence of the head of the navicular and the sustentaculum tali on the medial border.
3. The 'burying' of the lateral malleolus in soft tissue.
4. The 'bowing' of the tendo calcaneus as it leaves its attachment to the rotated calcaneus (this being known as 'Helbing's Sign').

Here it is important to note that not one of these signs by itself indicates conclusively that the foot is in valgus.

Where the valgus inrolling of the foot is accompanied by arthritic changes or other factors which may indicate that correction cannot be achieved or the soft tissues re-educated to hold the foot in correction, a means must be found to alleviate pain due to stress. The usual way in which this is done with adhesive felt is to make a pad which will 'fill the gap', as it were, of the area which should not be weight-bearing. This pad will alleviate stress in the soft tissues by passively supporting the bony structures of the longitudinal arch, although it has its limitation in that it will not actively correct the deformity. In the type of case at present under discussion, active correction could not be obtained due to the changes which have occurred in the tissues. One of the early signs of the foot which is going into valgus is excessive perspiration due to pain resulting from stress and, at this stage, active correction is not yet required, but passive support will relieve the stress (and the hyperidrosis) sufficiently to allow the tissues to readjust themselves to normal weight-bearing. This kind of condition may be seen in the school-leaver or other person unaccustomed to pro-longed weight-bearing taking up a job which entails long hours of standing or walking.

Having confirmed the diagnosis and method of treatment with adhesive padding (although this last may not be possible where hyperidrosis is a factor), the next step is to produce a washable appliance which will fulfil all the functions of the adhesive pad without the disadvantage—in this case—of being attached to the skin.

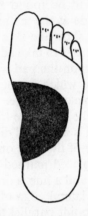

Fig. 62. A position for the valgus rest pad on the foot. Note how it 'fills in the gap' of the non-weight-bearing part of the plantar surface of the foot.

First, the position of the pad relative to the foot in the corrected position in the shoe must be made to appear on the insole pattern. The adhesive felt pad is cut to shape and put in place on the foot (Fig. 62), then the line formed by the lateral edge of the pad is marked *on the skin* with the ball-point pen (if any mark were to be made on the felt it would usually fail to transfer satisfactorily to the insole pattern), and no strapping is applied. Then the patient is asked to walk for a few minutes with the otherwise bare foot in the laced-up shoe and on the insole pattern, after which the position of the lateral edge of the pad on the corrected foot will be found to have transferred to the insole pattern. Had the pad not been worn at this stage, the resultant marking on the pattern would have been of no practical use because the foot would have been in valgus. The line of the edge of the pad as it appears on the template is then re-inforced by drawing over it with the ball-point pen and this one template with its line (together with the name and relevant details of the patient) is all the information that is required in the surgery.

Regenerated leather would be of little or no use as a base material for this appliance as it would be required to follow a number of curves in different planes, so $\frac{1}{16}$ in. closed cell split sponge rubber will be found to be one of the possible materials for a base having the additional advantage of being washable. The type of split sponge in $\frac{1}{16}$ in. thickness generally used as a base has much smaller cells in its closed cell construction than that used for padding; this has the effect of retaining the comparatively thin mass of its sheet in the shape to which it has been cut, and due to the greatly reduced size of the cells, it will be found more difficult to distinguish the skin from the cell side as the texture of both appear rather similar, but palpation will show the skin side as being 'smooth' and the cell side 'rough'. In order to take advantage of the increased traction of the cell side upon the pad which is stuck to it and upon the insole of the shoe which is not, the appliance is made so that this side faces the insole of the shoe.

In order to present an unbroken surface of the appliance to the foot, the base will lie *on top of the pad*, so there is a marked difference in the technique in marking out the shape of the base on the sheet of split sponge. The paper template is placed marked side uppermost on the skin side of the split rubber, and a line is drawn round its edge from the posterior end of the lateral edge of the pad (as marked), round the heel seating to a point parallel to it.

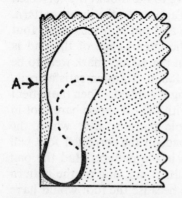

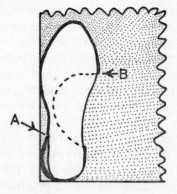

Fig. 63. The paper pattern (marked side uppermost) on the skin side of the split sponge; note the $\frac{1}{2}$ in. clearance (A) from the edge of the split sponge sheet. The heel part only is first outlined on the sponge as indicated by the thickened line.

Fig. 64. The paper pattern has been 'swung' through three degrees or so laterally (the $\frac{1}{2}$ in. clearance disappearing), and the outline is continued from the lateral end of the first outline (A) to point B.

(Fig. 63) Now, if the outline were to be continued from here without interruption, no allowance would have been made for the distortion of the base caused by placing the pad beneath it, so the index finger of the left hand is placed at the centre of the breast of the heel of the template and, using this as a fulcrum, the template is 'swung' laterally through about 3 degrees (or $\frac{1}{2}$ in. deviation of the anterior end from its original position), and the outline is continued forward along the lateral border, round the anterior edge and up to the anterior end of the pad (as marked). (A to B in Fig. 64) The paper template is now taken away to reveal the outline of the insole base *without* the section of the medial border where it coincides with the pad. Since the medial edge of the pad will form an *outward* curve in order to follow the contour of the longitudinal arch, and there being no accurate method of measuring it, it is necessary to find some arbitrary way of describing it on the gap in the outline. So the paper pattern is turned over and placed so that the marks for the anterior and posterior ends of the pad coincide with the two ends of the gap in the insole outline, and the curve of the edge of the paper pattern—now an *outwards* curve, is marked in (Fig. 65), and the base as outlined is ready to be cut from the sheet of split sponge.

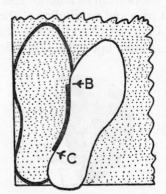

Fig. 65. The paper pattern, marked side now towards the split sponge, is placed so that the anterior end of the mark for the pad coincides with the mark at B, and the posterior end of the mark (C) for the pad (see also Fig. 64) coincides with the mark on the sponge. Then the pattern is outlined from B to C.

The next step is to use the template to derive the shape of the pad itself; here it will be recalled that the template bears only the line of the lateral edge of the pad, and this is now heavily inked in with the ball-point pen, the pattern turned over so that the marked side faces a clean sheet of paper beneath, and the unmarked side of the template is heavily scribbled upon over the area of the reinforced line, which will then transfer to the underlying paper. The template is now turned the right way up again and placed on the sheet of paper adjacent to the line which appears on it in a way which appears to make it run in a continuous ellipse. The edge of the paper pattern (which divides the ellipse) is now outlined, and when the pattern is taken away, the shape of the pad appears on the sheet of paper. The pattern for the pad is now cut from the sheet of paper, and besides marking it with the name of the patient, it will later be found useful if the word 'skin' or 'skin' side' (with an 'M' for medial at the medial edge of the pattern) is written on the under surface (with 'cell' on the top side of the pattern), which is now placed on the skin side of a sheet of ¼ in. closed cell sponge rubber so that the word 'Skin' appears uppermost on the pattern. The edges of the pattern are marked on the rubber and the pad is then cut out *but not skived* at this juncture. Now the thickness of material required along two-thirds of the length of the medial edge of the pad (before skiving) is ½ in. in most cases, so a smaller pad must be superimposed on the first, large one, in such a way that its medial edge coincides for the required two-thirds, and its lateral edge falls at the required distance short of the lateral edge of the large one. Starting at the point one-sixth of the total length of the medial edge of the pattern from its anterior end, a curve is drawn parallel to the lateral edge and concluding at the same distance from the posterior end of the pad. (A to B in Fig. 66) This smaller pattern is now cut out, placed upon the skin side

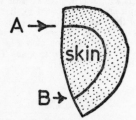

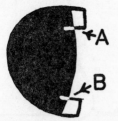

Fig. 66. The paper pattern is marked on its medial edge at points A and B, which are each about ⅙ of the length of the medial edge from the anterior and posterior ends, and a line is drawn from A to B parallel to the lateral edge of the pattern. Note that the word 'skin' appears on this, the underside of the pattern.

Fig. 67. The dark area represents the cell side of the larger pad, which is resting on the crescent-shaped off-cut of the paper pattern. Marks are made on the cell side of the larger pad at A and B to indicate the positions for the anterior and posterior ends of the medial edge of the smaller pad, which will be superimposed here after the two surfaces have been cleaned with rubber solution.

of the sheet of closed cell sponge rubber (the word 'Skin' on the pattern uppermost), outlined, and the pad cut out. Next, the cell side of the larger pad and the skin side of the smaller are cleaned with rubber solution, and when dry they are attached to each other in such a way that they will fall into the relative positions of the original pattern shown in the illustration (Fig. 66), and this may be achieved by placing the crescent-shaped off-cut from the larger pad pattern under the larger pad so that the two ends of the off-cut show at both anterior and posterior ends of the larger pad at its medial edge; the smaller pad is then positioned so that its medial edge, whilst coinciding with that of the larger pad, falls within the area indicated. (Fig. 67)

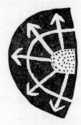

Fig. 68. The lighter area shows the remaining surface of full thickness from which the whole pad is skived right down to its lateral border.

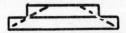

Fig. 69. The two pads, viewed in cross-section from the medial edge. The dotted lines show how the skiving will graduate the edges.

The two pads now being stuck firmly together, attention must be paid to the skiving on the cell side down to the lateral border of the 'sandwich' which will form one pad, because this is the surface which will be attached to the under side of the split rubber base. Accordingly, a mark is made on the exposed cell side of the smaller pad of roughly one-third of its length on the medial border, and a line is drawn parallel to its lateral border, this forming a guide from which the pad will be skived right down to the lateral border of the larger pad. (Fig. 68) At this stage the medial border of the pad remains unskived (Fig. 69), and the whole of the top surface of the pad is cleaned with rubber solution, together with an area of the under side of the base material, both being laid aside to dry.

The paper pattern of the insole of the shoe bears a mark showing the position of the pad in relation to the insole, so when the rubber solution is dry, the *pad* is placed on the *paper pattern* of the insole so that its lateral edge coincides with the mark on the pattern (its medial edge, of course, will not conform to that of the insole of the shoe, and will overlap and obscure that of the underlying paper pattern). Leaving the pad resting in the position described, the split rubber insole base is held (skin side uppermost) over both pad and paper pattern, and the posterior and lateral edges of the heel first placed in such a way as to touch those of the pattern, the lateral border only of the base is now rolled on to that of the pattern, and in this way the base is re-swung so that it just allows for the inclusion of the underlying pad whilst conforming to the shape of the insole of the shoe.

The top surface of the appliance is now complete, but underneath the full thickness of the pad extends right to the medial edge of the base material at the section which will rest on the side of the shoe. So it is necessary to relate the exact extent of the flat insole of the shoe to this surface of the appliance, and this is done by placing the appliance on the work bench with its under side uppermost, placing the insole pattern on top so that its posterior, lateral and anterior borders coincide with those of the base, and drawing an outline of the edge of the pattern on the pad. This line gives the starting point for the underskiving, which extends from here to the medial edge of the split rubber. (Fig. 70)

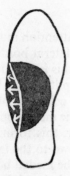

Fig. 70. On the underside of the appliance the skiving extends in the direction of the arrows, from the mark indicating the medial edge of the insole of the shoe to the medial edge of the base.

Thus the insole base has been re-swung to conform to the insole of the shoe, and the pad has been positioned to conform to that found satisfactory in adhesive padding on the corrected foot, conforming to its degree of defect; but being fairly soft and supple, the appliance *depends* almost entirely *on the shoe* for its success.

The shoe must be a strong lace-up type, as otherwise the action of the foot on the appliance will stretch the shoe out of shape. This appliance is called a valgus rest pad. It is no more than that.

7. 'CHAIRSIDE' APPLIANCES

'Chairside' appliances may be defined as removable appliances of fairly durable materials (such as leather and rubber) which may be made in the surgery in the presence of the patient, using the living foot upon which to measure and finally place them. The method of construction must be quick and comparatively clean, and the materials must be kept to hand. Thus this kind of appliance is a quick and simple one.

In order to provide the appropriate materials in a state of readiness, some preparation is necessary. In the section on adhesives it was shown that leather and other porous, non-rubber surfaces must be coated with latex, allowed to dry and kept clean before they will stick either together or to any other rubber surface satisfactorily. The leather most often used in this work is one of the suède splits (such as gas meter skin) and since the pieces required will be small off-cuts or 'roundings', these are saved up during normal appliance work, brushed with latex and immediately placed wet side downwards on to a sheet of clean polythene, the air being pressed outwards from the centre of the leather. The result will be a collection of roundings of differing size and shape, one side of each having a clean rubber surface from which air has been excluded. These roundings may be kept in this condition for very many months until they are needed in the surgery. The materials required for chairside appliances will be:

1. The polythene sheet with prepared pieces of gas meter skin.
2. Open and closed cell sponge rubber of different thicknesses.
3. A tin of rubber solution.

The pads themselves are a matter for the judgement and experience of the chiropodist as to what shape, size, thickness, position and type of adhesive padding has proved most beneficial in the past. It is possible to produce most digital pads, from a 'Dudley Morton' prop to a crescent for the fifth toe, using this method as long as complete conformity of the appliance to the detailed shape of the toe is not required, in which case it would be necessary to take a plaster cast of the part and use an entirely different technique. To discuss the two examples already mentioned should provide an adequate starting point from which to discover how to make any chairside appliance.

1. The Removable 'Dudley Morton' Prop

Having investigated the condition thoroughly to find that a 'Dudley Morton' prop is the requisite treatment, and that the patient is sufficiently agile and intelligent to use a removable one, the procedure is first to cut out the pad and underskive it all round, marking the positions for the toe loop attachments to the skin (or non-skived) side, and then cleaning the cell side with rubber solution after having measured the required length for the toe loop. Here the position of the loop relative to the pad and toe should be noted; on the lateral edge of the pad, the loop leaves the edge of the pad at a point about one-third of the length of the proximal phalanx from its head, passes interdigitally so that its folded edge will rest comfortably in the webbing, over the dorsum of the proximal phalanx, and finds attachment to the medial edge of the pad at the level of the *base* of the proximal phalanx. (Fig. 71) This position will be found useful since it *prevents the pad from moving—*

1. Backwards, because of the loop in the webbing.
2. Laterally, because of the attachment at the base of the proximal phalanx.
3. Medially, because the shoe itself will prevent this.
4. In a twisting movement, because of reasons 2 and 3.

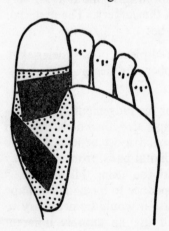

Fig. 71. The black areas on the 'Dudley Morton' prop show the positions and extent of the anchoring tabs for the toe loop.

The prepared cell side of the pad, when dry, is placed on to the rubberised dry surface of the gas meter off-cut, which is then trimmed round to within ⅛ in. of all the edges of the pad. The loop for the toe, which has been prepared in much the same manner as that for a metatarsal pad except that its adhesive surface is already treated with latex (Figs. 30 and 31) is then placed in the position marked on the pad, after which the top surfaces of its anchoring tabs are cleaned with rubber solution. Here there is an apparent anomaly; a leather surface is being cleaned with rubber solution instead of being coated with latex, and although this is not ideal it will give quite good anchorage since the main strain will occur between the tab and the pad, not the tab and its cover. Whilst cleaning the anchoring tabs with rubber solution, then, the whole of the skin side of the pad is treated in the same way, so that when the rubber solution is dry the final cover may be placed in position and trimmed round, thus completing the appliance.

2. The Crescent Pad for the Fifth Toe

The patient who has of necessity to wear a crescent for a corn on the fifth toe, caused by pressure from shoes which may be a hard-won compromise between what would be suitable and what is fashionable, could be an example of the right kind of case for a chairside appliance, although it does not follow that the cause of any corn can only be unsuitable shoes. Such a patient, if she persists with the shoes, will be condemned to a protective crescent on the toe until the fashions change to an unprecedented extent. Failure on the part of the chiropodist to accommodate the wishes of the patient by supplying suitable protection will result in a worsening of the condition, which would give rise to such pain that a change of gait and ultimately of posture would result, leading to the setting up of further painful conditions, together with a steady deterioration in the state of health of the foot and perhaps worse. The patient who is determined to put up with anything, whatever the cost and in the face of expert advice, to satisfy the whims of fashion and appearance is unhappily well known to every practitioner. The need then, for a more permanent form of protection than adhesive padding is well established, and this kind of patient particularly would welcome something which will assist her to maintain a higher standard of hygiene than she has hitherto found to be commensurate with comfort. These remarks could be applied to many a useful appliance, one of which is where a 'Dudley Morton' prop is being used in its removable form to relieve overloading of the 2nd and sometimes the 3rd and 4th metatarsal heads caused by the backthrust on the 2nd, 3rd and 4th toes making the 2nd, 3rd and 4th metatarso-phalangeal joint areas take more than their fair share of the load due to the constant wearing of court-type shoes. The answer, of course, rests with footwear, but the professional model or the ballet dancer is hardly in a position to be able to take this advice without seriously affecting her means of livelihood, and here the removable 'Dudley Morton' prop will be found to afford considerable relief from the symptoms.

The crescent for the 5th toe, then, is made as a chairside appliance by first cutting out the pad, skiving it on the cell side, and cleaning the *skin* side with rubber solution after measuring off the required length, and marking the positions of the attachments of the toe loop. Since this pad is a *dorsal* digital one, the skiving *faces the upper* of the shoe (which is not a flat surface). The toe loop, in this instance, will pass between the 4th and 5th toes. The rest of the procedure is the same as that described for a chairside 'Dudley Morton' prop.

From these two examples, it will be seen that most of such digital padding that is flat lends itself to translation to chairside appliances as long as the patient is able to manage them, and the same principles of construction apply to all of them. If, during the construction process, the prepared surface of the leather has been inadvertently handled, it is easily cleaned with rubber solution to restore it to its original condition of a clean rubber surface. The polythene sheet with the prepared pieces of gas meter roundings is kept in an accessible and cool place in the surgery, but during times when appliance work other than that of the chairside type is being carried out, it is useful to coat any off-cuts with latex and place them immediately in blank spaces on the sheet in order to avoid the embarrassment of finding none of suitable size when required.

CHAPTER V

MATERIALS USED IN CASTING

Plaster of Paris

Plaster of Paris is the material used for the positive cast. It occurs naturally as Calcium Sulphate Dihydrate (or 'Gypsum') which was first mined near Paris. The natural substance is roasted to a temperature of 130 deg. C. to convert it to Calcium Sulphate Hemihydrate $CaSO_4.\frac{1}{2}H_2O$, an amorphous powder which, when water is added, will convert back to the dihydrate $CaSO_4.2H_2O$ which is crystalline in structure. The Calcium Sulphate *Hemi*hydrate is the powder to which water is added, when the layers of powder which are in contact with the water will become supersaturated before the lower layers, which will in their turn convert to the dihydrate; so it will be seen that *time* is taken for the complete conversion. Should the hemihydrate be left undisturbed in water, the crystals in the resultant dihydrate will be large and therefore brittle, but if the mixture is stirred during the conversion stage, the crystals will be small and the dihydrate strong in comparison. Thus a given amount of hemihydrate will use only a certain amount of water—the water of crystallisation—and no more: this may be calculated by adding up the atomic weights of each so:

Calcium Sulphate *Di*hydrate			Calcium Sulphate *Hemi*hydrate		
	40	..	Ca ..	..	40
	32	..	S ..	..	32
	64	..	O_4 ..	..	64
$2H_2$ ..	4	..	.. $\frac{1}{2}H_2$ ..		1
2O ..	32	..	.. $\frac{1}{2}O$ ..		8
	172				145

So 27 of water in proportion to 145 should be required to convert the hemihydrate to the dihydrate, but in practice, much more water is needed and it will be found that (to use cookery proportions) 1 pint of water will take up 2 lb. of hemihydrate. In volume, as a

97

rule of thumb, it will be found that the amount of water required for a cast is roughly that of the volume of the cast itself, but it should be noted that the hemihydrate should be added to the water, *not* water to the hemihydrate. During the process of conversion there is an exchange of heat, but since the dihydrate is a poor conductor of heat there is no danger of burning the skin. In theory, discarded casts of dihydrate could be roasted at a temperature of 130 deg. C. and thereby be converted back to hemihydrate powder, but in practice this is never done due to the inconvenience of the operation and the apparent cheapness of the material.

Thus the plaster of paris powder is a material which, when water is added, will take and set in the exact shape of its container (faithfully reproducing any irregularities) to a hard dry substance which can be handled with ease, almost ideal for making life-size models of the foot or parts of the foot. The setting process is a chemical one (the conversion of the hemihydrate, by the addition of the water of crystallisation, to the dihydrate), not a physical one of merely drying out; this may be proved by adding a little of the hemihydrate powder to a large quantity of water, when the powder will only use its water of crystallisation to set quite hard at the bottom of the container *under water*. When the mix has been poured into the negative mould, the rubber bowl in which it was mixed should not be cleaned out until any residue of plaster has set, when it may be cracked out by turning the bowl inside out, waste plaster being placed in a bin, so avoiding choking up the drain of the sink. It is advisable, when using plaster of paris, to use a sink which has a plaster trap rather than one with the more conventional U-shaped drain trap which will easily clog up with plaster and periodically cause quite a major job for the plumber. Since the hemihydrate powder has an affinity for water, it should be kept in a dry atmosphere in an airtight container with the lid firmly on; when handling it, a parting agent such as soft soap should be used on the hands, paying special attention to the fingernails, because plaster of paris is difficult to remove from these areas unless this simple precaution is observed.

Plaster of Paris as an Impression Material. Plaster of paris used to be used as an impression material for practically any cast, including those now produced by using the resin and the alginate compounds or dental wax, but it still has its uses in this field as, for instance, in 'box' casting, or the taking of a whole foot cast. Due to its size and weight, a cast of the whole foot is not easily supported in these other materials, and plaster of paris will be found quite simple to handle for this operation.

Plaster of Paris Bandage. Although plaster of paris may be used by itself for taking a mould (or negative impression), it is often found to be too clumsy—too thick in the confined spaces of the toes, inconvenient and messy in proportion to the size of the task in hand in the surgery: thus various alternatives have been developed to obviate these difficulties. One of these is plaster of paris bandage, which basically is white open wove cotton bandage impregnated with plaster of paris powder (the hemihydrate). To reduce the tendency for the plaster to be lost from the bandage during wetting and handling, a technique has been developed which involves the manufacturers incorporating some inert resin which forms a jelly during immersion in water, thus holding the mass together. This type of plaster of paris bandage is known as 'Low Plaster Loss', or, 'L.P.L.' plaster of paris bandage. The material is used three or four layers thick, and since the hemihydrate powder is involved, care is taken to use the parting agent both on the hands of the operator and on the skin of the patient before commencing the technique.

The Resin Impression Compounds

There are a number of these compounds on the market which may vary in colour, but they are all made of resin with a filler—probably chalk—added. The material is supplied in slabs of $\frac{1}{8}$ in. to $\frac{1}{4}$ in. in thickness, and feels quite hard to the touch; if knocked reasonably vigorously, the slab will break, but the main advantage of this type of material is that it may be used over and over again for casting, since it polymerises (changes its state) so very slowly. Its action is a physical one—when placed in hot (not boiling) water, the resin softens and the slab becomes pliable, easily made thinner or longer and wider and so on, but more important, easy to mould to curved surfaces, when, if left to cool, the resin will begin to set again, although this time in the shape to which it was moulded. After the cast has set within a negative mould of this material, the impression compound may be removed by soaking the cast and the negative together in hot water, removing the softened compound, and rolling it out into a sheet again on a clean flat surface.

The Alginate Impression Compounds

This type of impression compound is also manufactured and supplied under different trade names and may vary in colour, but its essential composition is much the same. This compound is in a very fine powder form; the powder is an alginate derived from seaweed, and when mixed with the correct amount of water it forms a colloidal gel or jelly-like, almost rubbery mass which will retain its shape (although gradually undergoing slight contraction in size) for some time if kept in the correct conditions. As an impression-taking material it has the advantage of comparatively easy removal from the lesser toes even when they are quite badly distorted, together with producing a very highly detailed positive cast. It is quick and easy to use, but as the powder undergoes an irreversible physical change in use it is expensive—especially when compared with the resin compounds; thus it is only used in circumstances where either great detail is required in the positive cast or where it would be impractical to use a resin compound or plaster of paris.

Dental Wax

Dental wax is a useful impression material for digital casting, although the largest impression it will take is that of the first toe and its metatarso-phalangeal joint. It has the advantages of being quite cheap as well as able to be re-used a number of times, it involves the use of water which is warm rather than hot, and it moulds quite easily to complex curves, but its main disadvantage is that it is difficult to remove from any of the middle three toes without distorting the negative. In application, it will be found to be very clean (in this respect like the resin impression compounds), requiring water at a temperature of about 46 deg. C. to soften it, and there is no mixing of ingredients involved at the impression-taking stage. The form in which it is supplied—thin sheets—is easily cracked when cool, but this can be remedied by merely placing the cracked sheet in warm water and re-forming it.

CHAPTER VI

METHODS USED IN CASTING

1. BOX CASTING

THIS is a method, using *Plaster of Paris*, by means of which a cast of the whole foot may be obtained, although its principles may be applied to arriving at digital casts. It is essential that this process should be carried out where there is plenty of running water and a sink with a plaster trap, and care should be taken to cover the floor either with a large sheet of polythene or with old newspapers, as plaster is liable to be splashed about during the proceedings. The materials required to hand are:

1. A rubber mixing bowl.
2. Parting agent (soft soap).
3. Two pieces of string, 18 in. to 2 ft.
4. A shoe box of adequate size to leave good clearance all round the foot.
5. A good supply of plaster of paris.
6. Soap and towel, with a footbath.

Procedure. First the foot, and the hands of the operator, are carefully smeared with parting agent, paying special attention to the folds of the skin and to the areas round the nails. Soft soap is used as the parting agent in preference to petroleum jelly, for instance, as some of the parting agent almost invariably is transferred via the mould to the positive cast and thence to the appliance and since oil and rubber do not agree, soft soap will be found to be less damaging. Next, some plaster of paris is mixed in the bowl until there is sufficient to pour into the bottom of the shoe box and make it about one-third full. Mention has already been made about adding the hemihydrate powder to the water and using roughly the volume of water which is equivalent to the volume of plaster of paris mix required. The hemihydrate powder should be added to the water until it forms an 'island' which occupies about two-thirds of the surface area of the water, then stirring takes place to accelerate the chemical action and obtain smaller crystals of the dihydrate, until the consistency of the mix is such that the spatula can begin to stand on its own at an angle in the bowl, this indicating that the mix is ready to be poured. With the shoe box one-third full of the mix, then, the foot is placed in so that all its widest parts are just immersed to halfway (the toes, the 1st and 5th metatarso-phalangeal joint areas, the lateral border of the foot, and the whole of the heel area); the area under the medial longitudinal arch will have to be built up with plaster of paris until it reaches the base of the first metatarsal, the medial cuneiform, the navicular, the head of the talus, and slopes down again to the heel at its widest part. (Fig. 72) The foot is held quite still until the mix is solid, and then it is taken away and given more parting agent. Parting agent is now smeared evenly all over the upper surface of the plaster of paris 'footprint' in the shoe box, as well as all over the upper edges of the surrounding 'walls' of plaster.

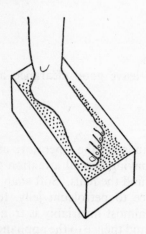

Fig. 72. The foot in the first mix of plaster of paris (the shaded area), the plaster reaching just as far as the widest parts of the foot and toes.

The two pieces of string are now placed on the foot, one starting above the ankle at its anterior aspect, passing down the dorsum of the foot and along the dorsum of the longest toe, leaving spare string at the end of the toe, whilst the other starts at the posterior aspect of the ankle, passing down the course of the tendo calcaneum and leaving ample spare string at the end where it will pass along the surface of the 'wall' of plaster and over the end of the box. With the string in position, then, the foot is replaced into its footprint in the shoebox, and the ends of the string are led up the ends of the shoebox and over the edges. More plaster of paris mix is now made ready and is poured into the box to cover the 'walls' of the first mix (which have been thinly coated with parting agent), the dorsum of the foot and the sides and posterior aspect of the heel, the mix covering these areas to a depth of two inches or so. When this has begun to set, the strings are both pulled gently out, one after the other, to divide the top shell longitudinally into two parts which, when properly set, may be removed separately after tearing away the sides of the shoebox.

The mould for the box cast now consists of three parts, two upper and one base. The foot and the operator's hands are washed free of plaster of paris, the mixing bowl, the floor covering, the parting agent and so on are cleared away before treatment is commenced.

Later, all the jointing surfaces, as well as the whole of the inner surface of the mould are covered with a fresh thin layer of parting agent, and the three sections are placed together and then securely tied together with strong string. Since box casting is relatively rarely called for, it is unlikely that there will be a rubber bowl available of sufficient size to take the appropriate quantity of mix to form the whole cast in one operation, so some fast working is called for. The first mix is poured in steadily and evenly, agitated so that it forms a thin skin of plaster all over the inner surface of the mould, poured back into the mixing bowl and then back again into the mould, taking care that air bubbles do not develop by allowing the mould to fill from the toe and by tilting it slightly forward. The next mix follows immediately until the mould is filled right up to the brim with the mix. The importance of care over the tilting during steady pouring cannot be over-emphasised, as air bubbles turn out as holes in the cast. The mould is then laid aside to set.

After twenty minutes to half an hour has elapsed, the securing string round the three sections of the mould may be removed and the sections taken away one by one, leaving a complete foot cast with small ridges of plaster (which may be smoothed out with emery cloth) along the lines of the joints of the mould. At this stage the cast will be quite warm, even though cold water was used for the mix, because of the heat generated by the chemical action of the conversion of the hemihydrate powder into the dihydrate cast. The chemical reaction will go on for some considerable time, but the heat is only generated during the early stages.

2. SLIPPER CASTING

A slipper cast, as the name suggests, is a cast of approximately that area of the foot which would be covered by the average carpet slipper, and the material used to take the impression is *plaster of paris bandage*.

The foot is first inspected to see that it is clean and free from grease or open lesions—a precaution always observed when taking impressions. The object is to make most of the length of the negative three layers of bandage in thickness, so, to avoid bending the dry plaster of paris bandage too much or too frequently (resulting in unnecessary loss of the hemihydrate powder), a length of 6 in. wide L.P.L. plaster of paris bandage is measured on the foot *from* the ball of the foot, up and into the longitudinal arch, round the heel *to* the attachment of the tendo calcaneus, leaving about ¼ in. to spare. (Fig. 73) This represents approximately half of one length of bandage required for the negative, so *double this length* is found, and then *three times* the double length will yield the full length of bandage required for the negative. This is cut from the roll of bandage and placed carefully aside on a dry, clean surface, the roll of bandage being wrapped up again in its grease-proof paper before being accidentally damaged either by too much handling or by moisture or wet plaster being splashed on it during the next processes. The foot and the hands of the operator are now prepared with parting agent, the floor beneath the plinth or leg-rest having been covered with a protective covering to catch the splashes or drips of plaster. A rubber mixing

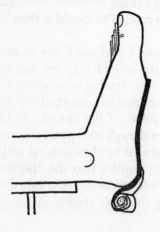

Fig. 73. One half of one length of dry plaster of paris bandage is measured against the foot as shown.

bowl about three-quarter full of water is placed conveniently near to the foot, and the measured length of plaster of paris bandage is folded into three, the two ends of the triple thickness being held between the second and third, and the third and fourth fingers respectively of one hand. (Fig. 74) The remainder of the length of bandage now suspended is rolled up loosely and gently and is lowered into the water in the rubber bowl, removing it again when it is just wet. With the other hand, the roll of bandage is squeezed very gently over the rubber bowl (just sufficiently to

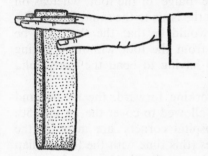

Fig. 74. The two ends of the triple thickness of plaster of paris bandage are held between the 2nd and 3rd and 3rd and 4th fingers of one hand as shown, before the free end is rolled up loosely.

remove excess water without extracting too much plaster of paris), and one end of the triple thickness is placed over the toes to be out of the way whilst the posterior end is receiving attention.

The posterior end of the triple thickness is now placed centrally or at about ¼ in. proximal to the attachment of the tendo calcaneum or at the point of the heel which projects furthest posteriorly (Fig. 75) and is folded back as far as the projection to form a reinforced edge of six thicknesses of bandage. This edge is carried

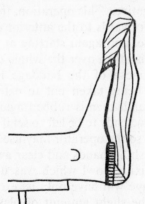

Fig. 75. The plaster of paris bandage in position for a slipper cast of the foot. Note the reinforced edges at the heel and at the dorsal metatarso-phalangeal areas, also the 'hospital corners' at the heel and toe.

round on the medial and lateral borders of the heel at its widest points so that the width of the bandage extends as a reinforced edge from the medial to the lateral borders of the heel. This edge is now smoothed against the skin and a 'hospital corner' formed with the bandage which will pass mainly along the plantar surface of the foot so that its edges fold upwards, and the material is laid so that it passes from the heel without wrinkling and that sufficient width is left to work up into the longitudinal arch. On the lateral border of the foot the edges of the bandage should come no higher than the most lateral edge of the 'bulge' of the foot, whereas on the medial side this will not affect the issue to the same extent. The result of ignoring this caution would be that the shell will be particularly difficult to remove from the foot without cracking due to the distortion caused by having to bend the fairly solid edges.

From the ball of the foot working forward, the medial and lateral edges of the bandage are allowed to cover the 1st and 5th metatarso-phalangeal joints, 'hospital corners' are made at the distal ends of the 1st and 5th toes (this time with the fold or flap extending *down* from the dorsum), over the distal ends of the toes and along the dorsal surface to a point just proximal to the heads of the 1st and 5th metatarsals, where any surplus bandage—there should be $\frac{1}{4}$ in. or more—is folded back to give a reinforced edge. (Fig. 75)

The next stage is to go back over the whole casting area, smoothing out any air trapped between the bandage and the skin and working from the heel along the mid-line of the foot towards the medial and lateral borders, 'herring-bone' fashion, squeezing air bubbles out of the sides of the negative. This operation, then, starts at the heel and works steadily forwards to the anterior end of the cast. When this has been done, and again starting at the heel, a gentle circular rubbing action is taken over the whole cast to 'cream' the plaster through the mesh of the bandage into intimate contact with the skin, care being taken not to extract more plaster by rubbing it on to the hands than is rubbed against the skin of the foot. The mould is now ready to be left to set if no correction is to be applied to the foot, so the operator may use the few minutes now at his disposal to wash his hands and clear away the floor covering. Note that the mixing bowl which was used for wetting the plaster of paris bandage will have only its excess water thrown away down the sink, the slight amount of plaster at the bottom of the bowl will be left to set, the remainder of the water then being poured away whilst the residue of plaster is cracked out and disposed of in the waste bin before cleaning the bowl thoroughly—this latter being done after the patient has left the surgery.

When the plaster negative has set, the skin near all its edges is moved so that air is allowed to enter between it and the mould. It will be remembered that the whole of the mould—with three parts of it excepted—is quite thin consisting of only three layers of plaster of paris bandage, and therefore comparatively easily fractured if subjected to much pressure or distortion. The three exceptions were those parts where 'hospital corner' folds were made, the posterior end of the bandage and the anterior end, both of which were reinforced to facilitate removal of the mould from the foot. At this stage, then, air having been allowed to enter between the mould and the foot, the fingers of one hand press downwards on the posterior reinforced edge whilst the other hand steadies the forefoot, the patient being asked to keep the foot as relaxed as possible. This movement should be a steady (not a sudden) one, and it continues just long enough to ease the edges of the posterior end of the shell clear of the plantar surface of the heel, when attention is transferred to the anterior reinforced edge, to which first a gentle rocking motion (to free the toes) is applied and then a forward and slightly sideways steady pull—one similar to that used for removing a slipper from the foot. The shell should now come quite readily away from the foot and should be examined for flaws or defects such as cracking caused by pushing the cast off the forefoot from the heel (giving buckling), or large air bubbles having been present, giving rise to areas inside the shell which will not have taken on the impression of skin wrinkles, which would result in bulges of extra material on the positive cast. If these or any other are sufficiently serious, the shell must be discarded and a second impression taken, going right through the process again with greater attention to detail.

Since these negatives are fragile, they are awkward to store, but as long as they are laid carefully out of the way of the possibility of accidental knocks or bumps, they will keep their shapes indefinitely; as this is usually inconvenient it is better to cast the shell as soon as possible.

The mould is filled to the brim with clean water, which is then emptied into a clean rubber mixing bowl. This quantity of water, it will be recalled, represents approximately that required to make about the same volume of dihydrate. The inside of the shell is now rinsed out with parting agent (soap solution) and the negative left, open side downwards, to drain.

The hemihydrate powder is now mixed with the measured quantity of water in the manner described previously for the mixing of plaster of paris until it approaches the desired consistency, when a little of it is poured into the mould, swilled round until the whole of its inside surface has a light coating of it, and the excess poured back into the mix in the bowl. The object of this exercise is to form a film of plaster of paris over the whole of what will be the surface of the positive cast in case air bubbles are accidentally formed in the main pouring—in which case they will now form *under* the surface of the cast. When the mix in the rubber bowl reaches the correct consistency, the mould is held in one hand with its anterior end inclined forwards and downwards whilst the even, creamy mix is poured steadily but gently in (to avoid air bubbles) until it reaches the anterior reinforced edge. A very short pause to let this begin to solidify, then the mould is tilted slowly back to the horizontal position whilst pouring in the rest of the mix. The whole is now placed in a tray of sand, which should be heaped up under the longitudinal arch to provide even support to the mould while the weight of the positive cast within is setting.

After not less than about twenty minutes, the hemihydrate will have been converted to the dihydrate and the cast will be set. It may be warm to the touch, even damp, but the shell may be removed as the cast will be no more set when dry than it will be at this stage. Removal of the negative from the cast will be found to be quite simple due to the 'hospital corners' which were made during the taking of the impression. There were four of these corners. Each is located and—with the help of the sharp point of the scissors working with the blade nearly horizontal to the cast—raised and unfolded. The toe and heel areas will thus be uncovered and the negative may be stripped from the cast and discarded.

3. DIGITAL CASTING

1. With Resin Compounds

A cast may be required only to show a hallux valgus (the toe, the joint, and approximately half the length of the first metatarsal). The resin compounds are particularly suitable as casting material for this sort of work, as there is ample room for manoeuvre. The slab of impression compound is placed in a bowl of very hot water, and the foot is seen to be clean and free from grease. When the compound has become easily and smoothly pliable, it is removed from the hot water and moulded on to the joint, round the toe into the interdigital webbing and over the required areas of the dorsal and plantar aspects of the metatarso-phalangeal joint. Then it is allowed to cool, and when nearly cold, is removed from the foot. If it is inconvenient to make the cast immediately, it will be found useful to place the negative in a rubber mixing bowl of cold water to ensure that it will not lose its shape through accidental knocks or unintentional re-heating from a radiator or other source of heat. One of the big advantages of these impression compounds is that no parting agent is required either on the foot or on the hands of the operator, and another is the absence of messy processes in the presence of the patient.

When pouring the plaster of paris mix into the mould, at first a little of the mix is poured in and swilled round the whole of the inside as was done with the slipper cast—to provide a surface for the positive cast which is free of air bubbles and to give a good 'key' for the rest of the mix. The mould is held in one hand with its closed (toe) end pointing obliquely downwards as the mix is poured gently in, tilting it gradually until it points vertically downwards; again, this is done in this way to avoid trapping large air bubbles in odd corners. As the plaster begins to set, so the mould is tilted gradually back to an angle approaching the horizontal (as the rest of the mix is added) to take the shape of the proximal end of the cast of the joint and metatarsal area. At a later stage it may be found useful to have a rudimentary 'handle' for the cast, thus, just before the plaster finally sets, a wood-screw may be sunk into the material with about half of its length at the head projecting above the level of the plaster; the screw is then left undisturbed to set solidly in the plaster. After twenty minutes to half an hour the cast will have set, and the procedure is to soften up the impression compound by immersing cast and negative in hot water (there being no danger of damaging the dihydrate cast since it will not dissolve in water) and simply remove the softened negative from the cast. Whilst the compound is still soft and pliable, any plaster which may have become embedded into it is removed, the material is squeezed into something resembling its original slab, placed on a flat clean surface—such as a sheet of plate glass—and rolled out with a clean glass cylindrical object (a bottle, maybe) in much the same manner as a rolling pin is used for pastry. The compound is then allowed to cool and harden and will be stored ready for re-use. The main drawback to this impression-taking material is that it will be found to resist removal from the middle three toes (in cases where they are deformed) with the effect that either it has to be distorted to such an extent as to spoil the impression and defeat its object, or the impression must be taken in two halves (plantar and dorsal) which are later fitted together before pouring in the plaster of paris mix.

2. With Alginate Impression Compounds

The procedure for making the mix with alginate compounds is usually clearly outlined by the manufacturers as far as the quantity of water required and the time for mixing is concerned. Great care should be taken to observe these scrupulously; too little water will give a very stiff intractable mass; too much water will result in an unusable solution, not a jelly-like suspension; too much time spent in spatulating the mix will mean that it will set into the suspension before it is removed from the mixing bowl; too little time will give a lumpy, uneven negative. The makers usually supply two measures—one for water and one for powder—with each tin, and the instructions are for dental purposes, but if the quantities are doubled they will be found to provide just a little more than sufficient material for casting one of the lesser toes together with some of the metatarso-phalangeal joint area.

No parting agent other than a little water being required on the foot, which is first checked to see that it is clean and free from grease, the procedure is to shake the tin of the compound before removing the lid to make sure that the powder, being very fine, is evenly packed (not more dense at the bottom of the tin than the top) and thus that the scoop provided will contain the correct quantity for mixing. The water having been measured out and poured into a clean mixing bowl, the powder is added, spatulating vigorously and taking care to see that a paste of an even consistency is achieved at the time recommended—usually about one minute. At this stage, the paste consists of a solution of the alginate in water, although it appears to be a mixture not unlike that of butter and sugar. The mixture is now worked into a mass which is lifted out of the mixing bowl and pushed over the apex of the toe to be cast, holding the adjacent toes apart, down to the interdigital webbing, some of the mass being taken on to the dorsum as far as the metatarso-phalangeal joint and a little on to the plantar surface of the foot (far enough to show where the weight-bearing area begins). The mass, or solution of alginate, is now left in position for two or three minutes until it has set into a colloidal gel with a shape, so to speak, of its own. The colloidal gel mass will feel 'rubbery' to the touch; it is capable, if stretched once slightly, of returning to its original shape; but it will not withstand repeated or violent stretching, so the technique of removal from the foot is first to introduce air between the negative and the skin by lifting the edges of the mass and moving it gently, then to grasp it gently and slide it off the toe in one smooth movement, bearing in mind the shape of the individual toe as this is done. The mould is fragile, and may easily be distorted by pressure, so it is placed straight into a rubber mixing bowl nearly full of clean cold water until it can be cast.

Casting the alginate negative should not be left for more than a few hours because of shrinkage of the mould. The procedure is quite simple; no parting agent is required, but the gaps left in the negative by the proximal phalanges of the adjacent toes should be bridged with adhesive plaster so applied that no tension is used to distort the shape. The plaster of paris mix is then poured in the manner previously described and left to set with an appropriate 'handle' such as a woodscrew, set into it. It has been postulated that if the mould is left on the cast for any great length of time, shrinkage of the colloidal gel as it loses its water content by evaporation will crack the positive. Despite lack of evidence to prove this theory experimentally, it is perhaps wise to remove the negative (by merely pulling it off in pieces and washing off any awkward remaining pockets) quite soon after the plaster of paris has set.

3. With Plaster of Paris (a Bi-valve Technique)

To use plaster of paris as an impression material in digital casting is rare nowadays, but it may be done by making a tray or small box out of stiff brown paper in such a way that it has an open end and no lid; its width is a little more than that of the diameter of the toe at its widest point, the flap of the open end extending along the plantar surface of the foot and the two free ends of the sides positioned so that they will come up against the interdigital webbing. The toe to be cast, together with the adjacent toes, the interdigital webbing and the appropriate part of the plantar surface of the foot are all prepared with parting agent. The 'tray' is rather more than half filled with plaster of paris mix and held in position under and along the toe, taking care to see that the level of the mix coincides with the widest part of the 'overhang', as it were, of the toe along its length. When the mix has hardened sufficiently, its surface is given a thin film of soft soap, and fresh mix is placed over the dorsum of the toe and as far as the upper edges of the sides of the plantar section. When this has hardened, the two sections are moved separately, placed together again and secured with either string or adhesive strapping, and the casting procedure from then is essentially the same (on a smaller scale) as that for pouring a box cast, great care being taken to avoid trapping air bubbles in the process.

4. With Dental Wax

Although dental wax is fragile and can be quite difficult to handle due to its sensitivity to warmth and its thinness, it is delightfully clean in the surgery and all that is required in the presence of the patient is two bowls, one containing warm water, the other cold. This is a useful material for those unable to tolerate the higher temperatures required for the resin impression compounds. The foot being clean and free from grease, the amount of wax required to cover the area is estimated, cracked off a sheet and placed on the surface of the warm water; while it softens, the appropriate part of the foot is moistened with some of the water. As soon as the sheet is sufficiently mouldable, it is removed from the water and placed on the foot, moulded over and round any prominences, and worked round the toe. Care should be taken not to overstretch any one part of the wax as this may thin it out too much to give a good impression, or it may even fracture the surface of the wax. The point at which the two edges meet on the medial or lateral border of the toe is that where they are turned back against each other, and will form a valuable identification place later in the procedure. The wax is left to set in this position as it cools, and the rate of cooling may be expedited by splashing cold water on it.

At the stage where the wax is nearly cold but still has a slight degree of pliability left, the two edges are opened out about half an inch, the mould is withdrawn from the toe and the edges repositioned immediately. The negative is then placed straight into the cold water to keep it at a comparatively low temperature and away from accidental damage until required for casting. It will be found advisable to keep the hands cold when handling the wax after it has been moulded to the toe to avoid distorting it with fingers otherwise possibly rather warm from the warm water.

Before casting the wax mould its free edges (interdigital and at the apex of the toe) must be sealed where they meet. The simplest way of doing this is to use adhesive strapping with no tension on it; a more sophisticated though delicate way is to warm the edges carefully with a lighted match so that they melt together and unite, but great care must be taken not to either overheat the wax and set fire to the mould or to allow the heat to reach other parts of the negative and distort it. The plaster of paris mix is then poured in the same way as for other digital casts (no parting agent being necessary), and when set, the cast may be removed from the mould by immersion in warm water and the wax may be retained for future use by preparing it in much the same manner as that used for resin impression compounds.

CHAPTER VII

CASTING TECHNIQUES

1. A CELASTIC VALGUS REST APPLIANCE

It will be recalled that the simple valgus rest appliance in split sponge rubber was one which completely relied on the shoe for its effect; without an adequate lace-up shoe on which it could exert some pressure it could not fulfil its function. The valgus rest pad relieved strain of the soft tissues of the foot by 'filling the space' between the longitudinal arch and the 'ground', and also relieved pain in the joints (in arthritic conditions) in two ways:

1. By limiting movement in the joints.
2. By redistributing compressive stress from the heel and meta-tarso-phalangeal joint areas.

To overcome the reliance of the fairly soft, space-filling pad on the shoe, a stiffer material is required; one which will exhibit four characteristics:

1. It must resist change of volume, so having a high modulus of compression.
2. It must resist change of shape, having a high modulus of rigidity.
3. It must be able to return to its original length when stretched, so having a fairly high modulus of elasticity, leaving some 'spring' in the foot.
4. It must be easily mouldable during construction.

Celastic ('Samcoforma') is a material which fulfils these requirements. Made of a cotton wove material impregnated with cellulose acetate—which gives it a fine granular surface—celastic is made in various thicknesses and grades, the one which has been found most useful in this work being graded S.B.120. This is a light grey material, and is supplied in sheets not unlike cardboard to the touch. Easily cut to shape with scissors, the material is then soaked in a suitable solvent such as ethyl acetate or acetone (which is more rarely used because of the high toxicity of its fumes), when the granules soften into a jelly-like mass; the wet material is then placed in position in the shoe or on the cast of the foot and is hammered lightly to compact the fibres of the material with the cellulose acetate and to eliminate gas bubbles. When the material has dried out, it will be found to be much harder and firmer than it was before treatment, and it may still be reduced and smoothed with the abrasive wheel if necessary. This material may also be built up in thickness layer by layer since cellulose acetate is quite a good glue, and indeed in some shoes celastic is used as a stiffener for the counters. Thus it will be seen that celastic fulfils the requirements outlined above.

To form the basis on which to make the appliance, a slipper cast of the foot which is set to show the pitch of the foot *in relation to the shoes* normally worn will be required, and this cast must be modified before the appliance is made.

The Pitch of the Foot. Very broadly, the pitch of the foot is the minimum height of the heel from the ground (when the ball of the foot is on contact with the ground and the leg is perpendicular) for the foot to be ready to work. A way in which to find the pitch of a foot with the patient seated is first to see that the tibia is horizontal or parallel to the floor by adjusting the leg rest and leaving the foot free. One hand is placed cupping the posterior border of the heel, with the index finger on the tendo calcaneus towards its insertion and the third finger on the posterior weight-bearing edge of the heel, the fourth and fifth fingers being free of the foot. The patient is asked to relax the foot and leg, the toes are grasped with the other hand which now dorsiflexes the foot until the tendo calcaneum is felt to begin to tighten and the forefoot starts to swing into supination; the foot is held in this position so that the transverse area of the metatarso-phalangeal joints will be seen to be parallel (or in the same transverse plane) to that of the heel. Now if the operator looks past the ball of the foot perpendicularly to the ground, he will not be able to see the heel, but he will be able to see one or more of the 'free' fingers of his other hand. The distance from the perpendicular (or part of the 'free' finger visible to the operator and closest to the heel) to the heel is a measurement of the pitch of the foot. (Fig. 76) This, then, is the pitch or angle at which the foot is mechanically ready to perform or function: a mobile valgus foot is capable of being swung into this position, and if it were possible to ensure its being so placed either during standing or when the body weight begins to be transmitted forwards from the heel, then conditions of comparative

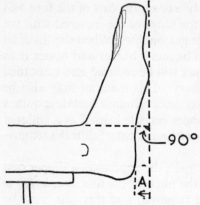

90°

Fig. 76. With the tibia parallel to the ground, the tendo calcaneum just beginning to tighten and the forefoot starting to swing into supination, the distance A is the pitch of the foot. Turn the diagram so that the foot appears to be standing on the ground, and it will be seen that this is the minimum height of heel which should be worn.

mechanical normality would have been set up. The celastic valgus rest appliance attempts to do just this, although it should be clearly understood that this is a rest appliance rather than a corrective one.

The procedure is commenced by taking a slipper cast of the foot in the position corrected for pitch at the stage where the plaster of paris bandage is just beginning to set. Here it should be remembered that the pitch imposed on the cast is that of the agreed height of heel of the shoe to be worn by the patient, not that of the foot. The pitch of the foot will first have been observed and noted, and taking into account that this is the minimum height of heel which should be worn, discussion with the patient in regard to the height of heel should yield a compromise between good and common sense, and it is this compromise which is imposed upon the cast, always remembering that the pitch *of the foot* represents the minimum height of the shoe heel to be worn. Whilst the patient is still in the surgery, a paper pattern of the insole of the shoe for which the appliance is designed is taken, and a mark made on the heel part of this to indicate the posterior point of contact of the plantar surface of the heel with the shoe (shown by the wear mark): although a detail, this information will be found to be vital towards the completion stage of the fabrication of the appliance. After the mould has been removed from the foot, it is examined for flaws and later cast.

When the foot is placed upon the ground and takes weight, it alters the shape of its soft tissues. So far as the purpose for which this cast was made is concerned, the relevant aspect of this change of shape is that of the soft tissues of the weight-bearing portions (with the exception of the toes) of the plantar surface. The degree to which these soft tissues become compressed is evidenced by a line or ridge (on the skin) which runs round the medial, posterior and lateral borders of the heel, is sometimes seen to continue anteriorly along the lateral border of the foot, and again becomes well defined on the lateral border of the 5th metatarso-phalangeal joint. On the medial border, the line is seen again at the edge of the metatarso-phalangeal joint. Since the base of the appliance is to be transversely flat (to conform to the flat insole of the shoe), the *cast must be modified* and this indicating line is the *key to the modification*. The parts of the cast directly relevant to the appliance all include, transversely, the whole of the plantar surface of the foot from the heel to the neck of all the metatarsals:

1. The plantar surface of the heel area.
2. The whole of the longitudinal arch 'space' to the neck of the 1st metatarsal.
3. The lateral border of the foot from the heel to the neck of the 5th metatarsal.

The cast is of the foot set for the pitch of the shoe, so it follows that areas 1 and 3, whilst being parallel to or in the same transverse plane as each other, will be on different levels, just as two steps may be in the same transverse (though in this case, longitudinally inclined at different angles) plane as each other but at varying levels.

Having determined the outline of the line of compression of the soft tissues, the cast is modified by transversely rasping, filing or abrading the heel area and the area of the metatarso-phalangeal joints from the medial line to the lateral line, thus removing plaster of paris from the cast and leaving flattened areas in both regions connected by the 'bridge', as it were, of the weight-bearing lateral border of the foot. Attention is now turned to this 'bridge', finding the compression line and rasping from lateral to medial in a transverse plane parallel to that of the heel and forefoot, thus leaving the gap (resembling in shape that of the letter D) representing the longitudinal arch space, unmodified. (Fig. 77) Next, the skin markings are removed from the longitudinal arch area by rubbing with emery cloth, and the whole of the required surface of the cast is treated similarly to remove any marks or indentations which would otherwise be reflected in the celastic of the appliance.

It will be necessary, by using layers or laminations of celastic, to build up the thickness and strength of the appliance in much the same way as a leaf spring, under the longitudinal arch. In this case, a total of four thicknesses are built up at the thickest part, one sufficing for the thinnest. Thus patterns must be devised for the different pieces of celastic, and since they will be designed to cover curved areas, special steps must be taken to ensure their correct fit.

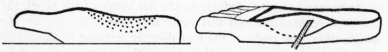

Fig. 77. A medial view of a slipper cast of the left foot, set for the pitch of the shoe. The light shading represents the area of the medial longitudinal arch.

Fig. 78. A postero-medial view of the cast, the thickened lines indicating the modified edges of the plantar surface, with the chalk travelling anteriorly along the medial edge at an angle of 45 degrees to the transverse plane.

Using coloured chalk, the outline of the largest and first layer of celastic is drawn on the cast, particular attention being paid to the medial border which, if it is too low, will not perform its function adequately and if too high, will be at such an angle as to cause the soft tissues of the foot to fold or 'lip' over it, the edge biting in, causing pain to the patient, and such undue stress on the material that it will tend to give way. Since the heel and forefoot are parallel to the transverse plane of the shoe and ground, a line on the cast following a contour at 45 deg. to the transverse plane would describe an arc as it travelled forwards and this would be the line of the highest point of the medial border of the appliance. Thus this line is chalked on the cast by holding the piece of chalk at an angle of 45 deg. to the transverse plane of the heel and fore-foot and, starting at the heel, allowing the chalk to contact the medial border of the cast and drawing it forwards to the first metatarsal head. (Fig. 78) From this point, the chalk mark is taken across the ball of the foot to the fifth metatarsal head, posteriorly along the flattened edge (at the compression line) of the modified plantar surface of the cast, round the heel, and so joining up with the posterior end of the line starting on the medial border of the cast. The area now marked represents that of the first (longest) layer of celastic. Attention is now turned to the second layer.

With the cast held upside down so that the eye sees the medial border, and tilted until the transverse plane of the heel and fore-foot appear to form a single straight line or 'horizon' (as in Fig. 77), a chalk mark is made to start at the point where the first line or mark representing the medial edge of the appliance dips down from the 'horizon', along what appears to be the horizon until it reaches the first line again. (Fig. 78) This lateral line now represents the lateral border of the second layer, which is seen to cover the whole area of the space under the longitudinal arch. The medial border of the second layer is now divided into segments by first marking its highest point in relation to the ground, allowing for the pitch in the shoe (Point A in Fig. 79); thus it has been divided into two unequal lengths, each of which is now divided into thirds.

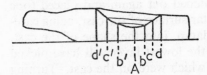

Fig. 79. At the anterior end, Ab equals bc which equals cd along the lower curve. The same applies at the posterior side of A, but the anterior sections are not equal to those of the posterior.

Again holding the cast upside down at eye level so that, looking at the medial border, the lateral border mark of the second layer appears as the 'horizon', starting at the most anterior of the marks just made on the medial border, a line is drawn to what will appear to be parallel to the 'horizon' until it meets the most posterior of the newly made division marks, thus making a line in the contour of the longitudinal arch space as seen in a contour map. (c/ to c, Fig. 79) This line, then, indicates the lateral border of the third layer, its medial border being shared with that of the first and second. The lateral border of the fourth layer is marked by joining the outside two of the remaining three marks. (b/ to b, Fig. 79) The anterior and posterior ends of the second, third and fourth layers should now have lines drawn from them up the medial side of the cast and at right angles to the 'ground'; these will serve as indicators when the pattern of lines is obscured by the first layer of celastic.

The cast, then, is now marked up with the outlines of the edges of the laminations or leaves, and the next step is to transfer these markings (Fig. 80) to paper in order to arrive at paper patterns for each layer. Newspaper is used, and to facilitate moulding to the curved surfaces, it is first thoroughly soaked in water. Thus four layers of newspaper are together soaked in water, the excess water

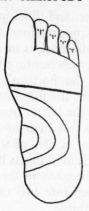

Fig. 80. A plantar view of the marked slipper cast. The anterior transverse line comes just posterior to the metatarsal heads, and note that the marks for the posterior ends of the leaves are closer together than those of the anterior ends. See also Fig. 79.

squeezed out, the layers straightened out again and placed (one on top of the other) on the plantar surface of the cast, being careful to mould them whilst still damp, into the shape of the cast. When the papers are removed, the lowest layer will have picked up some of the chalk markings which were on the cast. Turning them over so that the marked layer is uppermost and keeping all four layers of newspaper together, they should be cut to the shape of the largest outline in chalk, the bottom layer of paper (which now nearly represents the shape of the first layer of celastic) being taken from the other three and laid to one side. Next, the outline of the second layer is cut out, and the bottom layer of paper taken from the other two and laid to one side. The process is repeated for the third layer, and the fourth already is marked on the remaining layer.

All four paper patterns may now be allowed to dry out, and the cast is soaked for a few minutes in water, taken out and given a thin coating of special parting agent and after an interval of five minutes a second coat of parting agent is applied. The four paper patterns are used to cut out the desired shapes of celastic, but here it should be observed that whilst the patterns of the second, third and fourth layers should be closely adhered to, that of the first should not—a spare ½ in. or so should be left on the lateral border, and on the posterior border, the medial border only being taken as the shape of the pattern dictates. (Fig. 81)

The four celastic shapes are next placed in a shallow tray containing sufficient ethyl acetate to cover the bottom, and the fingers of the operator are moistened with the special parting agent supplied by the manufacturers of celastic. The largest, or first, shape

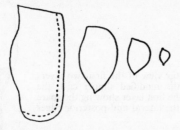

Fig. 81. A general idea of the shapes of the paper patterns for the laminations. The dotted line on the largest indicates where spare celastic is allowed at the posterior and lateral edges.

is now placed on the prepared cast (so that its medial and anterior borders coincide with those marked) and moulded to the contours of the underlying plantar and medial aspects of the cast. When this is done, the whole of that portion of the shape in contact with the cast is tapped with the fitter's hammer to compound the cellulose acetate with the cotton fibre mesh and to eliminate any pockets of gas which may have accumulated whilst the celastic was in the solvent. The second shape is now positioned so that its anterior and posterior pointed edges coincide with the outside two perpendicular lines (on the medial edge of the cast) and its medial edge falls just short of the medial edge of the first layer. (Figs. 82 and 83) This is then tapped with the fitter's hammer and the edges smoothed as far as possible to merge with the first layer. The same procedure is followed for the third and fourth layers, the whole is bound lightly to the cast with bandaging to retain its shape while it is left to dry.

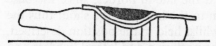

Fig. 82. A medial view of the first two layers of celastic in position on the modified slipper cast. See also Fig. 83.

When the celastic has dried thoroughly, both it and the bandaging is removed from the cast. The shape of the celastic on the medial border was a result of careful calculations and markings, so it may therefore be regarded as being accurate, whereas that of the lateral and posterior borders was allowed to be oversize and will have curled up round these borders of the cast, setting in this shape, so it is now hammered lightly on its under side until it lies continuous with the transverse planes of the cast.

The dry celastic shape is next laid in position on the cast and the

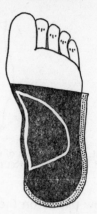

Fig. 83. A plantar view of the first two layers of celastic on the modified slipper cast, the lighter area on the first layer showing the spare material left at the lateral and posterior edges See also Fig 82.

paper pattern of the insole of the shoe is placed on top of it with its marked side towards the cast. The mark ('A' in Fig. 84) indicating the point of contact of the heel of the foot with the heel of the insole pattern is made to coincide with the point of contact of the heel of the modified cast with the celastic, and the medial border of the pattern to coincide with the medial edge of the celastic at the heel and at the first metatarsal head area. (Fig. 84)

A

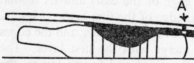

Fig. 84. A medial view of the paper insole pattern resting on the celastic. The mark (A) on the insole pattern is aligned with the point of contact of the heel of the cast with the celastic, the surplus of which (projecting beyond the insole pattern) is trimmed off. See also Fig. 85.

Some celastic material will then be seen to be superfluous to requirements at the heel and at the lateral border, since the base of the appliance must conform to the insole of the shoe; thus the outline of the paper pattern, whilst held in the position described, is marked on the celastic at the posterior and lateral borders and the excess material trimmed off. (Fig. 85)

Since covering leathers will be employed, paper patterns are taken of the shape and area of both the upper and lower surfaces of the celastic mould (this may be done with either crêpe paper or with wet newspaper so that they may mould to the curves presented), and each pattern is marked to indicate its purpose. The top surface of the mould is now coated with latex and allowed to dry whilst the covering leathers are being prepared.

The leather selected for the top surface should be a grain one,

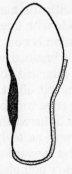

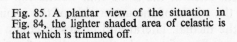

Fig. 85. A plantar view of the situation in Fig. 84, the lighter shaded area of celastic is that which is trimmed off.

able to withstand quite hard wear. Persian lamb or glacé kid would be obvious choices. First the paper pattern is used by outlining it (with about half an inch to spare all round) on the flesh side of the leather selected, then, from the resulting leather shape, ¾ in. is skived from the flesh to the grain side of the medial, lateral and posterior edges to facilitate turning over these edges of the celastic. The whole of the flesh side of the shape is now coated with latex and laid aside to dry, and since the top surface of the celastic base will be dry by then, it is turned over and the under side is treated with latex.

When the surfaces are dry, the covering leather is attached to the upper surface of the base, first at the highest point in the medial longitudinal arch area (leaving the skived edge free) and passing the cover gently into place from the point of attachment and across to the lateral border in a fanwise direction to follow the concave curve of the surface of the celastic. This fanwise attaching process is continued until the whole of the cover material is attached to the upper surface of the mould, leaving the skived edges free of the base.

At the medial and lateral corners at the anterior edge of the celastic, cuts are made, and the medial and lateral flaps are moulded over to find attachment to the under side of the base, but special steps must be taken at the heel area, due to its curvature. Here the leather must be pleated in much the same way as that used for the medial border of the cover of a 'Dudley Morton' Prop on an insole base. Starting by attaching the middle of the heel area with the back of a blade of a pair of scissors, then half-way between this and the medial border, then half-way between it and the lateral border, then dividing each section in half, and so on until it is impossible to go any further, finishing off by hammering lightly with the mallet and coating the top of the cover on the under side with latex.

Attention is now turned to the plantar covering material, which has been brushed with latex at the same time as the top cover. This is attached to the whole of the under side of the appliance and trimmed off at the medial, lateral and posterior edges. The anterior edge will form a flap of grain leather, to the under side of which is adhered the gas meter skin; this is now underskived in such a way as to have only about $\frac{1}{8}$ in. of the skived material projecting forward of the anterior edge of celastic, and the appliance is now complete.

In cases where, perhaps, a metatarsal pad, or one combined with a 'Dudley Morton' Prop or, indeed, where any pad is desired to be incorporated at the anterior end of the appliance, this may be done by making due markings (on the insole pattern of the shoe) from the foot of the patient, attaching the pad to the upper surface of the celastic in the position indicated on the pattern, and allowing the appropriate amount of extra covering material.

2. A CORRECTIVE VALGUS INSOLE

The types of valgus appliances previously discussed have had rest as their function. To obtain correction, the material used must not compress easily and must resist change of shape (so having a high modulus of Bulk or Compression and a high modulus of Rigidity); preferably, though not essentially, the material should also be easy to work, resistant to water and light in weight. Such a material is cork bottom filler.

Cork Bottom Filler

So called, because it is material used for 'filling the bottoms' of shoes during manufacture, cork bottom filler consists of granulated cork bonded with cellulose acetate—both of which are solids and will not compress easily—which is stiff and brittle when it is dry and set, and will resist change of shape. The cellulose acetate may be softened with a solvent—acetone—and in this softened, wet state, the material is 'puddingy' in consistency and easily spread with a spatula. Both cork and cellulose acetate are light in weight and resistant to water, although neither is very hardwearing, so it is placed in a position where it will not be subjected to much wear. The material is supplied in tins which should always be kept upside down because the granulated cork will float in the acetone; when the tin is inverted for use, air is allowed to enter, some of the acetone will evaporate and some dry granulated cork and cellulose acetate will be left on the inside of the lid and upper edges of the tin, and when the tin is turned upside down again, this material will be preserved.

Shoes. To work properly, the corrective appliance must be in a strong shoe which is a good fit, and of the lace-up type, coming over the tuberosity of the navicular; the heel stiffener must be adequate and come well forward, whilst the height of the heel must be no lower than the pitch of the foot.

Procedure

A paper pattern is taken of the insole of the shoe in the manner described earlier, and this is marked for the posterior point of contact of the heel (as for the celastic valgus rest appliance). A slipper cast of the foot in the corrected position is taken—marking the area of the sustentaculum tali. The resultant appliance will achieve over-correction of the foot by applying pressure to the area under the sustentaculum tali by the calcaneo-navicular or 'Spring' ligament. This will effect a withdrawal reflex, which re-educates the muscles by means of a modification to the cast to be described. If the muscles are paralysed, the withdrawal reflex will not be obtained, and the appliance will work only as a palliative support and cause a pressure sore under the area of the sustentaculum tali.

Cast Modification

As with the slipper cast for the celastic valgus rest appliance, the cast is modified by removing the bulge representing soft tissue up to the compression lines on the lateral, posterior and parts of the medial borders, but in addition the cast is excavated or deepened in the area of the medial longitudinal arch under the sustentaculum tali (as marked). For a thin, bony foot, the excavation is about ⅛ in. deep, for a well-padded foot, ¼ in.

Making the Appliance

First, a paper pattern is taken on the cast of the size of the top surface area of the appliance. This is carried out in a similar method to the way used for the celastic valgus rest appliance, making the highest point coincide with the mark on the cast for the sustentaculum tali and again taking care to leave extra allowance at the heel and lateral border of the foot. The material to be used as base upon which to build the appliance will again be celastic, and since the cellulose acetate dissolved in acetone is the cement in the cork bottom filler, a particularly good bond will occur with the celastic. The template is used to cut the celastic from the sheet, the cast is saturated in water and then given two coats of parting agent, then the celastic shape is wetted in ethyl acetate, placed in position on the cast and hammered with the fitter's hammer. Next, the bottom filler is spatulated on to the celastic, 'filling in the space', as it were, of the longitudinal arch slightly clear of the level of the insole of the shoe, little attempt being made at this stage to shape it accordingly. (Fig. 86) The incomplete appliance is then bandaged on to the cast (to help to retain its shape), and laid aside to dry out.

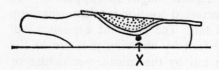

Fig. 86. A medial view of the corrective valgus rest appliance (before completion) on the excavated cast. The shaded area represents cork bottom filler in the longitudinal arch 'space', and 'X' is the mark for the sustentaculum tali.

When dry, the bandage is removed and the paper pattern of the insole of the shoe is placed in the position described for the celastic valgus rest appliance over the appliance, and its edges outlined on the appliance. The surplus cork bottom filler is then skived on the abrasive wheel from the mark to the medial edge of the celastic, this being done whilst the appliance is still on the cast and before its lateral and posterior edges have been modified (these having the effect of holding the appliance in position during skiving, the cast imparting some rigidity to the cork, which would crack if subjected to much bending at this stage). The appliance is now removed from the cast and after hammering the lateral and posterior edges of the celastic until they are flat, the surplus material is cut away, leaving the flat base of the appliance now conforming to the shape and size of the insole pattern of the shoe.

It remains now to cover the top and bottom of the appliance in suitable leathers, for instance, glacé kid and gas meter skin, and this is done in much the same way as the celastic valgus rest appliance, and the appliance is now complete. When the foot brings pressure to bear on the area under the sustentaculum tali, a withdrawal reflex will operate, causing the muscles to contract (re-forming the arch) and re-educating them to hold the foot in its proper position.

3. A VALGUS REST MOCASSIN

Both the celastic valgus rest and the corrective valgus insole appliances, whilst differing from each other in action, depended upon and were made for one particular shoe or pair of shoes; neither could be worn in any shoe other than that for which it was made, but there are cases where, for instance, a valgus rest appliance is required which can be worn in any of a number of different shoes, in which case a valgus rest mocassin would be a suitable choice of appliance.

The procedure is to make a slipper cast of the foot in the position where both transverse planes of the metatarsal and calacaneal areas are parallel and the foot is adjusted to its own pitch (not the pitch of the shoe, since the appliance is designed to go into any shoe). No modification is made to the cast other than a smoothing out of the skin striations, and the next step is to take about half a dozen strips of white open wove bandage, each of a sufficient length to cover an area from the metatarso-phalangeal joints to about half an inch posterior to the weight-bearing surface of the heel, placing them flat on a sheet of glass, brushing them with latex and leaving them to dry.

A piece of split suède—gas meter skin—large enough to cover the whole slipper cast excepting most of the dorsal surface is cut out and punched with a leather punch about $\frac{1}{2}$ in. all round from the edges, and using these holes, the leather is sewn with string (criss-crossing the dorsal surface of the cast) under tension in such a way as to stretch it over the whole of the plantar surface with as few wrinkles round the edge as possible, and none at all on the plantar surface. A second piece of split suède of slightly smaller dimensions is cut out, and both are coated with latex and put aside to dry. A piece of $\frac{1}{16}$ in. closed cell split sponge may then be adhered to the plantar surface, sufficient to cover the weight-bearing area from the necks of the metatarsals, into the longi-tudinal arch and back to the heel. Now the pad—in this case, the valgus rest pad—is cut out of closed cell sponge rubber, built up to the required thickness and skived on the cell side so that the skin side will come next to the cast. The skin side is then cleaned with rubber solution, and when dry it is placed in position on the prepared surface of the leather which is stretched over the cast, then the skived cell side is cleaned with rubber solution.

The prepared strips of bandage, which will act as reinforcing material to help the appliance keep its shape, are now stripped from the glass sheet and laid from the metatarso-phalangeal joint area to just posterior to the weight-bearing surface of the heel, each overlapping its neighbour and so that together they cover the width of the plantar surface of the appliance and about ½ in. over the medial and lateral borders of the rubber. Care is taken to see that the reinforcing strips are not wrinkled, and are in firm contact with the underlying surface of the rubber or the gas meter skin, and the whole surface is then cleaned with rubber solution.

The second piece of prepared split suède is now placed over the appliance and allowed to contact and adhere to it, confining any wrinkles in its surface to above the edges of the reinforcing strips, and pressing well down over the whole of this final cover to give good adhesion. The appliance can now be cut from the cast, trimmed round all the edges to ⅛ in. of the reinforcing strips and it is complete.

4. DIGITAL APPLIANCES, WITH A LATEX DIP TECHNIQUE

This is a technique which was largely developed for use in chiropody by J. W. J. Turvey, M.Ch.S. (see *The Chiropodist*, Vol. XI, September 1956, p. 267) and results in appliances which will fit the toe intimately having had only two dips in centrifuged vulcanised latex. One of the alternative methods of producing virtually the same appliance is to dip the cast repeatedly in latex and allow it to dry between each immersion, thereby gradually building up the required thickness of rubber over a comparatively long period of time; quicker than this is the acid accelerator system (see *Chiropodial Orthopaedics*, by Franklin Charlesworth, F.Ch.S.) in which 10 per cent hydrochloric acid is used between each dip to obviate the time required for drying; but here again each layer has to be built up one upon the other, may quite easily contaminate the latex bath, and produces a weaker rubber film unless very considerable attention is paid to the neutralising and washing processes, which again take time.

The equipment necessary for this technique is as follows:

1. Two tanks for dipping, both of approximately the same size (large and deep enough to take the biggest cast which will be used whilst leaving at least half an inch to spare all round), one with an airtight lid to prevent evaporation of the stabiliser from the centrifuged latex. The second tank is for the coagulant salt solution.
2. An oven or drying cabinet, the temperature of which can be controlled and raised when required to 90 deg. C., and through which air can circulate.

The materials needed are:

1. 30 per cent coagulant salt solution (as supplied by Messrs. Revertex Ltd., who devised it).
2. 60 per cent centrifuged latex.
3. Closed and open cell padding material (rubber).
4. Rubber solution (with carbon tetrachloride as a solvent).

Method

An impression of the toe is taken, seeing that sufficient of the dorsum of the foot (in the case of an appliance for the dorsal surface) is cast to allow rather more than the necessary area upon which the pad will rest. The mould is cast, and after the impression material has been removed, the cast is examined for flaws such as pits in the surface left by air bubbles; if these exist, they may be filled up and smoothed off. Any rough edges or 'seams' are smoothed out with a knife or with emery cloth, and the cast is placed in the drying cabinet where, when it is completely dry, it is heated to a temperature of 60 deg. C.

The heated cast is removed from the drying cabinet and promptly dipped—for about half a second—in the coagulant salt solution, holding the cast by its 'handle' (a woodscrew being useful for the purpose), after which it is allowed to cool and dry off. When it is dry, a layer of fine crystals of the coagulant salt will be found to have formed just under the whole of the porous surface of the plaster. Next, the cast is dipped carefully into the centrifuged latex until it is completely immersed, where it is held or hung quite still for a period which will vary according to the thickness of rubber required for the first layer or film; the time is usually about two and a half minutes, after whch it is carefully removed, the end which went in first—the distal end—coming out first and seeing that the cast does not touch the sides of the dip tank. Whilst the cast was in the latex, the coagulant salt crystals just below its surface were causing the latex to 'gel' evenly over the whole of the area; had the cast been left in the bath indefinitely, the rubber gel would have become thicker and thicker until all the centrifuged latex had been used up, hence, by accurate timing, the ease and convenience of keeping control over the thickness of rubber is acquired.

The gel on the surface of the cast is inspected carefully for any flaws. Rapid dipping or withdrawal will cause air-bubbles; if these are few enough and small enough, they may sometimes be obliterated by carefully bursting them with a pin, though this may leave a pitted surface in the appliance. The precaution of skimming the surface of the centrifuged latex should be observed before starting a session of dipping, since any impurities in the air trapped between the lid and the surface of the latex may have precipitated on to the latex, and the surface will tend to be formed into a slight skin since some of the stabiliser will have inevitably evaporated into the trapped air (this is why it is important to keep the tank as full of latex as is practicable). Should the surface of the gel on the cast be spoiled, the gel itself may be quite easily removed by merely pulling it off, dipping the cast again in the latex. No further dipping in the coagulant salt will be necessary before doing this, as the crystals will have remained just below the surface of the cast.

The cast, with its gel, is now placed in the drying cabinet on a rack in such a way that the wet rubber will not come into contact with the shelves or with other appliances, at a commencing temperature of not more than 40 deg. C. in circulating air. While the gel is drying out, its cloudiness passing, it will change colour from white to a clear amber, the temperature of the cabinet may be gradually raised to 90 deg. C. to facilitate the drying process. As this is taking place, the pad may be prepared.

As an example, suppose a crescent for the fifth toe is required. The pad will be made of closed cell sponge rubber, cell side towards the foot. Special attention must be paid to the skiving, which must be carried out in such a way as to exert the minimum possible strain on the surface (the first layer of rubber) to which it is adhered. Here the contour of the surface of the cast will indicate where under- or over-skiving is required. An underskived edge which has to be 'bent down to' the surface to which it is to adhere will tend to lift the rubber from the cast, distorting the appliance, whereas an overskived edge which is bent up to conform to the underlying contour will exert no strain on the rubber film. With these considerations in mind, the pad is devised and prepared and very thoroughly cleaned (of any rubber dust which may have collected on it after skiving on the abrasive wheel), and its cell side is then cleaned with rubber solution.

When the gel is clear amber, the cast is removed from the drying cabinet and the pad is placed carefully in position, where it will stick instantly since the surface of the gel is clean rubber. If, however, the cast has remained in the drying cabinet for very much longer than necessary, dust might quite possibly have collected on its surface (especially as the oven is designed to allow the free circulation of warmed air), and if this is the case, an area slightly larger than that to which the pad will be attached is cleaned with rubber solution or with ether before the pad is applied. The cast, with its first film of rubber and the pad attached, is now returned to the oven and heated up to 60 deg. C. again; when this is done, it is again dipped in the coagulant salt solution for half a second, great care being taken not to handle the rubber surface in case the layer of coagulant salt crystals is wiped away. The exposed cell surface at the skived edges of the pad are blotted with some clean open cell sponge rubber to prevent a thicker layer of crystals (so ultimately, a thicker layer of rubber) forming here when the cast is cool and dry.

Next, the whole is dipped gently into the centrifuged latex and held quite still for as long as is required to build up the necessary thickness of rubber. The usual procedure is to use a total dipping time of five minutes, so if the first immersion was timed at two and a half minutes before applying the pad, the second will be another two and a half. The cast is gently removed in the same way as before, inspected for flaws, and put back in the drying oven at a commencing temperature of 40 deg. C., rising gently to 90 deg. C. as the cloudiness passes in the gel. When the rubber has become a clear amber, it is stripped from the cast after powdering the outside with talcum powder, and the excess rubber at the edges is trimmed off to the required shape. It is usually advisable to cut a hole in the region of the toenail, both for aeration of the skin and to leave the nail and sulcus free of any constriction.

At this stage, the dried latex sheet contains serum enmeshed within its substance which materially reduces its resilience and strength, so it is advisable to macerate or 'steep' the appliance in lukewarm water for not less than two hours—twenty-four or forty-eight hours is better still—to allow this to dissolve out, so increasing the durability and life of the appliance quite considerably.

The process, then, is quite simple. First, the cast of the toe is taken, dried out and the surfaces prepared, heated up, plunged into coagulant salt solution for half a second, allowed to dry and cool, held or hung in the centrifuged latex for two and a half minutes and warmed gently to dry whilst the pad is prepared. The pad attached, the whole is heated up again, dipped in the coagulant salt solution for the second time, allowed to dry and cool (the pad having been blotted), the whole dipped for the second and last two and a half minute dip in the centrifuged latex and warmed to dry, after which it is powdered, stripped from the cast and powdered on the inside, trimmed and macerated and allowed thereafter to dry out completely, when it is ready to wear.

This process is one of the few, the various stages of which can be carried out during five minute breaks in the appointment schedule of the busy private chiropodist; the longer intervals of the drying stages can be profitably put to use treating patients.

5.   DIGITAL APPLIANCES, A HALLUX VALGUS SHIELD

When a patient has an allergy to or a dislike of rubber, but some protection is required for, say, an H.V. joint, the latex dip technique is ruled out because it involves using rubber next to the skin and, depending on the degree of deformity, a chairside appliance would be unsuitable because it would not conform to the very marked contours of the area to be protected. In cases of this type, it is possible to produce an appliance which is covered in suède split, and although thicker than the latex dip type, will be found to conform to the foot in a very satisfactory manner and to be most comfortable and practical in use.

First, an impression of the toe, the joint and at least half the length of the metatarsal is taken either with one of the resin impression compounds or with dental wax. This is cast, the negative removed and the cast allowed to dry out very thoroughly before disposing of any unwanted 'seams' or ridges with either emery cloth or knife. Next, the cast is covered with gas meter skin stretched quite firmly over the whole of its area—with the exception of the toe area—in such a way that the ends of the skin may be drawn tightly together over where the open end of the mould was; these ends are attached under mild tension either with adhesive strapping or by sewing them together. The toe area may be dealt with by treating the inside of the opposing flaps (at the lateral border of the toe) with latex, allowing them to dry and pinching them together, trimming off excess material to give a butted join. A strip about half an inch wide on either side of the join is now brushed with latex, and when this is dry, a half-inch strip of white open wove bandage, which has previously been brushed with latex and allowed to dry, is placed lengthwise over the join to attach to the prepared surfaces on either side of the join, anchoring them together. (Fig. 87) The area of the leather to which the pad will be attached is now brushed with latex and allowed to dry.

The object of this pad is to protect the metatarso-phalangeal joint from pressure mainly from the anterior and posterior directions, with a slight degree of protection from the dorsal and plantar directions. To this end, the pad will be oval-shaped, having a recess or cavity into which the prominence of the joint will fit, the full thickness of the pad taking the burden of the pressure. Accordingly, the oval shape is cut from the sheet of closed cell sponge rubber, cleaned on its cell side with rubber

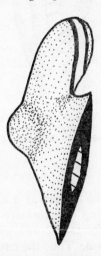

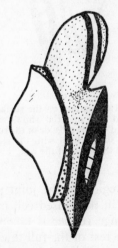

Fig. 87. The cast covered in split suède. The open end (heavily shaded) is where the leather is stitched or strapped together; the longitudinal lines on the toe area show where the rubberised strip of $\frac{1}{2}$ in. bandage is placed over the butted edges.

Fig. 88. The unskived closed cell sponge rubber in position.

solution and allowed to dry; no skiving or other preparation of the pad being carried out at this stage.

The cell side of the pad is now attached to the prepared surface of the gas meter skin on the cast, stretching the sponge rubber slightly before moulding it from the prominence of the joint to the surrounding areas in such a way that only that part of the pad which will form the cavity is under stretch. The situation now is that a piece of closed cell material, the edges of which conform to the shape of an H.V. oval, has been placed in position on the covered cast without any skiving or other modification at all; the full thickness extends over the whole area. (Fig. 88)

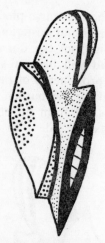
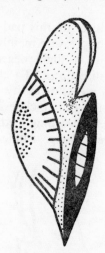

Fig. 89. The shading on the surface of the closed cell material shows where the 'mound' on the cell side of the rubber has been skived level with the surface of the full thickness of the rest.

Fig. 90. After skiving at the edges, the pad makes a smooth contour with the foot to present to the inside of the shoe.

The region of the joint prominence will appear as a lump or mound in the closed cell material so, using the abrasive wheel, the sponge rubber is taken off until it forms a continuous line with the rest of the full thickness of the pad. Thus the cavity has been formed by skiving on top of the pad, the slight stress on the rubber which was caused when moulding it to the joint prominence has been largely relieved, leaving a clean outside line and a smooth inside surface of the pad nearest to the foot. (Fig. 89) With the abrasive wheel, the edges of the pad are skived down to the edges

(Fig. 90) taking care not to buff the leather as well, the incomplete appliance is dusted to remove the rubber dust (from the skiving process), the pad itself is cleaned with rubber solution and the rest of the leather surface brushed with latex and allowed to dry.

Using more of the rubberised $\frac{1}{2}$ in. w.o.w. bandage, a strip is placed in the manner of a sling, starting on the pad, going round the toe and so back to the pad again (Fig. 91); this will serve to prevent distortion of the appliance in wear, as the leather would otherwise stretch so that the pad would eventually lie posterior to its proper position. The whole area is now covered with its final cover of gas meter skin, the edges of which are butted on the lateral side of the toe, the appliance is cut from the cast, the edges trimmed and an aperture cut for the toe-nail, and it is complete. (Fig. 92)

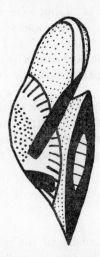

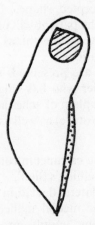

Fig. 91. The reinforcing strip of rubberised w.o.w. bandage (seen here in black), passing from the pad, across the dorsum, on the lateral side of the toe and so across the plantar surface to find anchorage on the pad again.

Fig. 92. With its aperture for the toe-nail, the appliance is complete.

CHAPTER VIII

MODIFICATION TO FOOTWEAR

A VALGUS STIFFENER

CHILDREN as patients present various conditions for the attention of the chiropodist. Babies and toddlers are brought to the surgery with the observation of the anxious parents that they have 'flat feet', 'bow legs' or 'knock knees', and it is now generally recognised that the 'flat feet' are not usually flat at all, but have not been used sufficiently yet to fulfil their normal function and so assume their accepted shape. Even in cases of 'bow legs' and 'knock knees', the patient will often grow out of the condition by the time he is seven or eight as long as there are no systemic or other complications.

Cases are presented, though, of the child of nine or ten or a little older who has valgus feet. This child will stand badly and may complain of aches and pains in various parts of the body (due to bad posture) as well as in the feet and legs. The signs of a valgus foot,

1. The calcaneum rotated so that its lateral border is raised,
2. 'Helbing's Sign',
3. A lateral deviation of the forefoot,
4. The medial malleolus and the tuberosity of the navicular being unduly prominent, whilst the lateral malleolus is partially obscured in the soft tissues.

are present, and the patient tends to 'break down' his shoes at the medial borders. Provided that there is no major muscular or similar defect, this is the kind of case where modification of suitable footwear over a reasonably short period of time will usually serve to have a corrective effect which will be permanent, the modification being discarded as the shoes are outgrown. The main advantage of modifying the shoes of a child of this age is that the child can neither remove it from the shoe nor lose it in his locker at school—there is, then, no valid excuse for the appliance not to be used. Also, incidentally, time is saved by obviating any necessity for a cast to be taken of the foot as in a corrective valgus insole appliance.

It is preferable to start with new lace-up shoes which, whilst a good fit, allow adequate room for growth. The shoe is put on the foot, inspected with these factors in mind, and the position of the sustentaculum tali in relation to the inside of the shoe is marked lightly: this point is usually over the breast of the heel. This is all that is required in the surgery.

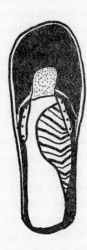

Fig. 93. A view of the paper pattern (the shaded area) in the shoe from which the lace has been removed.

A paper pattern is now devised (Fig. 93) the posterior end of which lies well back on the medial side of the calcaneum, its lateral border missing the medial tuberosity of the calcaneum, but swinging out laterally in front in something resembling the shape of the lateral border of the valgus rest pad, and swinging in again to the medial border of the insole of the shoe at the anterior end of its waist. The medial border of the paper pattern will describe an arc up the medial side of the shoe, the highest point lying just under the tuberosity of the navicular.

From this first pattern, two smaller ones will be derived, each about one-third smaller than its predecessor. Most shoes have a thin 'sock' covering the true insole, the material of which this is made depending on the price and quality of the shoe. This 'sock' is now carefully removed—it is usually only lightly stuck in—and the area of the inside of the shoe which is covered by the paper pattern is roughened with emery cloth and cleaned with ethyl acetate. Between the insole and the medial border of the upper there is a slight gap or trough. A long thin piece of celastic is wetted with ethyl acetate and tamped into the trough to fill it for the length of the distance between the anterior and posterior ends of the largest paper pattern.

Next, celastic is cut to the shape and size of the three paper patterns and placed in the tray containing a little ethyl acetate. Then they are placed in the shoe one by one, the smallest going in first, in such a way that the first piece has its middle on the mark, the successive pieces are superimposed so that more overlap occurs to the front, and the tail of the largest piece meets the beginning of the curve of the heel seat. Each piece is tamped down with the fitter's hammer as it is placed, and when dry any further smoothing off which may be necessary may be carried out with emery cloth.

Finally, the dry celastic may either be painted or covered with skiver leather, and the original 'sock' replaced in the shoe by first brushing its under side and the area with which it will come in contact with latex, and allowing the two surfaces to dry before bringing them together. The modification is then complete.

The effect of this modification is to cause a withdrawal reflex, making the muscles themselves correct the foot and so in time establishing a conditioned reflex. At first, then, the patient will be aware of discomfort when wearing the shoe, but not of his reaction to it. As the conditioned reflex is established, so the discomfort becomes less and less noticed until the patient can do without the modification and is able to maintain the arch without mechanical assistance.

CHAPTER IX
SUMMARY

FOR many years past much time and energy has been spent on making pads to which both the patient and the operator had become addicted; today an alternative is presented which can relieve the chiropodist of work which was routine and can often save the patient from becoming a 'chronic' case.

When the adhesive padding approach to a case has reached a stage of maintaining comfort and function without possibility of further improvement, and has therefore become a long-term treatment, an appliance may often present an attractive alternative since it will give more permanent correction, protection or cushioning, thereby preventing certain conditions from becoming chronic.

However, three factors were mentioned which must be considered before translating existing padding into appliances. The patient. The foot. The shoe. The patient must comprehend the purpose of the change in approach and be able to manage the appliance; co-operation is needed. The case selected must be carefully appraised to see that no alteration of adhesive padding is likely to improve the condition further—an appliance, after all, will neither fit the foot as intimately nor move with it so closely as the adhesive pad. The shoe must be adequate to accommodate the foot and to provide a basic structure complementary to the appliance. Without an appreciation of these factors, there is a likelihood of failure in the use of an appliance, with consequent loss of confidence on the part of both patient and operator in appliances as a therapeutic measure.

Certain basic types of appliances have been discussed in broad relationship to the conditions which they are designed to treat. Since the pads have been of open or closed cell sponge rubber, the adhesives, cover and base have been chosen as the most suitable to use together. The techniques employed in the fabrication of appliances have proved very satisfactory over a number of years but when the practitioner has become adept in appliance making he will no doubt find modifications without loss of accuracy so long as he has grasped the fundamental points stressed.

The principles expounded herein can be applied in the management of most foot disabilities. If a technique described in these pages suggests an alternative approach to the reader, let him pursue it, for that is the purpose of such an introduction. Techniques are being evolved for use with new materials such as the plastics and silicone rubbers, which may lead to appliances which can be constructed more quickly, but whatever the future may hold, the basis upon which the work is carried out must be sound and reasoned so that the beneficial effect to the patient presently achieved by the intelligent and thoughtful use of appliances may not only be preserved but also extended.

INDEX

141